CLASSROOM TRAINING HANDBOOK

NONDESTRUCTIVE TESTING

Ultrasonic

Published by *PH D*iversified, Inc.
5040-B Highway 49 South
Harrisburg, NC 28075
704-455-3717

Printed in the United States of America
ISBN 1-886630-16-X

PREFACE

Level II Classroom Training Handbook - Ultrasonic Testing, CT-4 is one in a series of training handbooks designed for basic Level II training when NDT is taught in a traditional classroom setting. The instructor would typically assign chapters and discuss the material in a classroom lecture format. To provide complete Level II classroom training the instructor should supplement this text with assignments that include industry specific applications and related practical examinations.

This Level II Classroom Training Handbook also serves as an excellent reference book during on-the-job training of nondestructive testing personnel.

This handbook is most effective when used by those persons who have successfully completed the **Level I Programmed Instruction Handbook, PI-4**, Ultrasonic Testing (3 volumes). The Programmed Instruction Handbooks present entry level material in a **self-study format**. A cross-reference guide is printed in this Level II Classroom Training Handbook so that the student can read corresponding information in the self-study handbook to provide a more structured approach for individual learning.

Other **Classroom Training Handbooks** in the series include:

CT-2   Liquid Penetrant Testing

CT-3   Magnetic Particle Testing

CT-5   Eddy Current Testing

CT-6   Radiographic Testing

It is recommended that PI-1, Introduction to Nondestructive Testing, be completed before starting this book in order to have the benefit of certain basic metallurgy information that will make this book easier to understand.

ACKNOWLEDGMENTS

Publishing and Printing

     Revision Editor: . . . . Dr. George Pherigo, *PH Di*versified, Inc.

     Production Editor . . Ms. Mary Lou Hollifield, *PH Di*versified, Inc.

     Proofreading . . . . Ms. Jean Pherigo, *PH Di*versified, Inc.
     Proofreading . . . . Ms. Dana Smilie

Technical Content Revision

     Technical Editor . . . . Mr. Robert W. Smilie

This handbook was originally prepared by the Convair Division of General Dynamics Corporation under contract to NASA and was identified as N68-28790. This book is part of a series of books, commonly known as the General Dynamics Series, that has been the basis of many industrial NDT training programs for over 20 years.

Now, after several decades of widespread use, the entire series has undergone a major revision. The revised material no longer concentrates on applications in the aerospace industry, but instead, covers a wider range of industrial applications and discusses the newest techniques and applications.

Mr. Robert W. Smilie has been the principal technical editor of the revised material in this text. Using his nondestructive testing experiences in several industries, including work at the EPRI NDE Center, he has updated the text to better suit the entry-level technician/engineer.

CLASSROOM TRAINING MANUAL
ULTRASONIC TESTING

TABLE OF CONTENTS

CROSS REFERENCE TO
PROGRAMMED INSTRUCTION HANDBOOKS

If this handbook is being used in a classrooom lecture format, the instructor may choose to make additional reading assignments from the Programmed Instruction series. The Programmed Instruction handbooks often provide a little more detail, especially in those areas that are most difficult to comprehend.

CT Text (Chapter & Page)	PI Text (Volume/Chapter/Page)
Chapter 1	N/A
Ch. 2: 2-1 to 2-4	Vol. I/Ch. 1; All: Ch. 3; 3-1 to 3-8
Ch. 2: 2-4 to 2-10	Vol. I/Ch. 3; 3-9 to 3-24, 3-43, 3-45
Ch. 2: 2-11 to 2-17	Vol. I/Ch. 2; All
Ch. 2: 2-18 to 2-27	Vol. I/Ch. 3; 3-26 to 3-49
Ch. 2: 2-27 to 2-32	Vol. I/Ch. 4; 4-1 to 4-9
Ch. 2: 2-33	Vol. I, Ch. 4, 4-10 to 4-27
	Vol. II, Ch. 5; All
Ch. 2: 2-34 to 2-39	Vol. I/Ch. 5; All
	Vol. III/Ch. 6; 6-20 to 6-35
Ch. 3: 3-1 to 3-14	Vol. II/Ch. 1
Ch. 3: 3-14 to 3-16	Vol. II/Ch. 2
Ch. 3: 3-17 to 3-23	Vol. II/Ch. 3
Ch. 3: 3-24 to 3-40	Vol. II/Ch. 4
Ch. 3: 3-41 to 3-43	Vol. II/Ch. 5
Ch. 4: 4-1 to 4-3	Vol. III/Ch. 1
Ch. 4: 4-3 to 4-8	Vol. III/Ch. 4
Ch. 4: 4-9 to 4-21	Vol. III/Ch. 1
Ch. 4: 4-22 to 4-30	Vol. III/Ch. 5 and Ch. 6
Ch. 4: 4-31 to 4-41	Vol. III/Ch. 2, Ch. 3; 3-1 to 3-70
Ch. 4: 4-42 to 4-48	Vol. III/Ch. 3; 3-71 to 3-92
Ch. 5	N/A

CHAPTER 1: INTRODUCTION

TABLE OF CONTENTS

CHAPTER 1

INTRODUCTION

General

The complexity and expense of today's machines, equipment, and tools dictate the use of fabrication and testing procedures that will ensure maximum reliability. Nondestructive testing (testing without destroying) provides many of these procedures. Of the number of nondestructive testing procedures available, ultrasonic testing - of which this handbook is concerned - is one of the most widely used.

Purpose

The purpose of this handbook is to provide the fundamental knowledge of ultrasonic testing required by quality assurance and test personnel to enable them to:

- ascertain that the proper test technique, or combination of techniques, is used to assure the quality of the finished product.

- interpret, evaluate, and make a sound decision as to the results of the test.

•   recognize those areas exhibiting doubtful test results that require either retest or assistance in interpretation and evaluation.

Description of Contents

•   Arrangement

The material contained in this handbook is presented in a logical sequence and consists of:

-    Chapter 1:   Introduction
-    Chapter 2:   Principles
-    Chapter 3:   Equipment
-    Chapter 4:   Technique and Applications
-    Chapter 5:   Calibrating Transducers
-    Appendix A: Comparison and Selection of NDT Processes
-    Appendix B: Glossary
-    Appendix C: Trigonometry Tables
-    Appendix D: Acoustic Properties of Materials

•   Locators

-    At the front of each chapter is a table of contents referencing the major paragraphs in that chapter. Also included is a list of figures and tables, where applicable.

Industrial Applications of Ultrasonic Testing

Because of the basic characteristics of ultrasonic testing, it is used to test a variety of both metallic and nonmetallic products such as welds, forgings, castings, sheet, tubing, plastics, ceramics, etc. Since ultrasonic testing is capable of economically revealing subsurface discontinuities (variations in material composition) in a variety of dissimilar materials, it is one of the most effective tools available to quality assurance personnel.

Testing Philosophy

Nondestructive testing is used to assure maximum reliability of machines, equipment and tools. To accomplish such reliability, test standards have been set and test results must meet these standards.

Personnel

It is imperative that personnel responsible for ultrasonic testing be trained and highly qualified with a technical understanding of the test equipment and materials, the item under test (specimen), and the test procedures. Quality assurance personnel must be equally qualified. To make optimum use of ultrasonic testing, personnel conducting tests must continually keep abreast of new developments. There is no substitute for knowledge.

Testing Criteria

Modern manufacturing procedures dictate that faulty articles be discovered as early in the manufacturing process as possible. This means that each item must be tested individually before it is required to perform in a subassembly and that each subassembly be tested before it is required to perform in an assembly, etc. This building-block approach requires that test processes be selected and test procedures be generated at the lowest level in the manufacturing process in order that the highest reliability may be obtained with lowest cost.

Test Procedures

Approved procedures for ultrasonic testing are formulated from analysis of the test specimen or article, review of its past history, experience on like or similar specimens, and information available concerning discontinuities in similar specimens. It is the responsibility of personnel conducting or checking tests to ensure that test procedures are adequately performed, and that the test objective is accomplished. Procedures found to be incorrect or inadequate must be brought to the attention of responsible supervision for correction and incorporation into revised procedures.

Test Objective

The objective of ultrasonic testing is to ensure product reliability by providing a means of:

- obtaining a visual recorded image related to a discontinuity in the specimen under test.
- disclosing the nature of the discontinuity without impairing the material.
- separating acceptable and unacceptable material in accordance with predetermined standards.

No test is successfully completed until an evaluation of the test results is made. Evaluation of test procedures and results requires understanding of the test objective as well as a knowledge of the material from which the test article is made. It also requires a knowledge of the manufacturing processes that were involved.

CHAPTER 2: PRINCIPLES

TABLE OF CONTENTS

TABLE OF CONTENTS (CONT'D.)

LIST OF FIGURES

LIST OF FIGURES (CONT'D.)

LIST OF TABLES

LIST OF TABLES (CONT'D.)

PRINCIPLES

Early Sonic Tests

For centuries, men tested parts by hitting them with a mallet and listening for a tonal quality difference. Around the turn of this century, railroad men inspected parts by applying kerosene to the part and covering it with a coat of whiting (chalk). In areas where the whiting looked wet, the part was assumed to be cracked. In the early 1940's, Dr. F. A. Firestone developed the first pulse-echo instrument for detecting deep-seated flaws. The establishment of basic standards and the development of the first practical immersion testing system are credited to W. C. Hitt and D. C. Erdman.

Ultrasonic Wave Generation

Ultrasound (or any frequency sound) is the mechanical vibration of particles in a medium (material). When a sound wave travels in a material, the particles in the material vibrate about a fixed point at the same frequency as the sound wave. The particles do not travel with the wave but only react to the energy of the wave. It is the energy of the wave that moves through the material. When a tuning fork is struck, it vibrates and produces sound waves by compressing the air. These waves travel through air to the ear of the listener as shown in Figure 2-1. The tuning fork vibrations soon die out and no longer produce waves. Similarly, in ultrasonic testing, a transducer (crystal) is electrically excited which then vibrates. The ultrasound from the transducer then travels through a couplant, which may be water, oil, etc., to the front surface of the test piece. Figure 2-2 shows the transducer in contact with the test piece and the ultrasound pulses traveling through the piece.

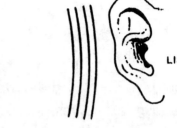

TUNING FORK

LISTENER

Figure 2-1. Sound Wave Generation

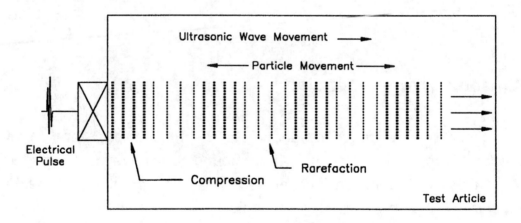

Figure 2-2. Ultrasonic Wave Generation

General

Ultrasonics is the name given to the study and application of sound waves having frequencies higher than those which the human ear can hear. Adults with normal hearing can hear frequencies in a range from 20 Hz to 20,000 kHz (thousand cycles per second). Ultrasonic nondestructive testing is the use of ultrasonics to examine or test material without destroying the material. An ultrasonic test may be used to measure the thickness of a material or to examine the internal structure of a material for possible discontinuities such as voids and/or cracks. Testing frequencies commonly range from 0.5 MHz (0.5 million hertz) to 25,000,000 Hz (25 MHz).

Modes of Vibration

If the length of a particular sound wave is measured from trough to trough, or from crest to crest, the distance is always the same. This distance is known as the wavelength (λ) and is defined in the following equation. The time it takes for the wave to travel a distance of one complete wavelength, λ, is the same amount of time it takes for the source to execute one complete vibration.

$$\lambda = \frac{V}{f}$$

Where:

λ = the wavelength of the wave

V = velocity

f = the frequency of the wave

Several types of sound waves travel through solid matter. There are longitudinal or compression waves where the particles vibrate back and forth in the same direction as the motion of the sound (as in Figure 2-2).

There are also shear or transverse waves where the particles vibrate back and forth in a direction that is at right angles to the motion of the sound. It is also possible, within certain limits, to produce waves that travel along the free boundary or surface of a solid.

These surface, or Rayleigh (pronounced "ray-lee"), waves penetrate the material to a depth of about one wavelength. Ultrasonic vibrations in liquids or gases are only propagated as longitudinal waves because of the absence of rigidity in liquids and gases. Longitudinal, shear, and surface waves can be propagated in solids.

The shortest ultrasonic wavelengths are of the order of magnitude of visible light. For this reason, ultrasonic wave vibrations possess properties very similar to those of light waves; i.e., they may be reflected, focused, and refracted.

The high frequency particle vibrations of ultrasound waves are propagated in homogeneous solid objects in the same manner as directed light beams. Ultrasound is reflected (partially or totally) at any surface acting as a boundary between the test object and a gas, liquid, or another type of solid. As with echo-sounding in sonar applications, the ultrasonic pulses reflect from discontinuities, thereby enabling detection of the presence and location of the discontinuity.

Wave Modes

- General

    All materials are made up of atoms (or tiny particles) lined up in straight lines to form lattices, as shown in Figure 2-3. If we strike the side of this lattice, we find that the first column of atoms strikes the second column rebounding and reverberating back and forth and striking the third column and so on in sequence. This particle motion produces a wave movement in the direction shown. In this case, the particle movement direction is the same as the wave movement direction. This type of ultrasound wave motion (or mode) is called the longitudinal or compression wave mode. This wave mode travels the fastest.

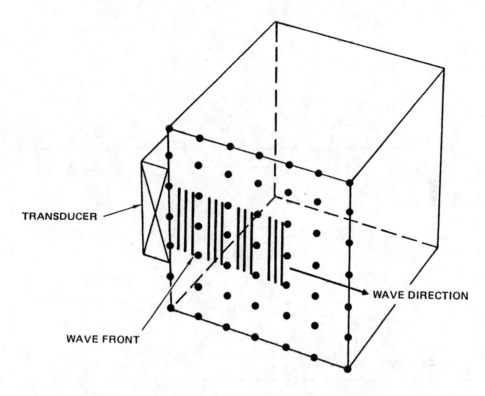

Figure 2-3. Longitudinal Wave Mode

● Comparison of Longitudinal and Shear Wave Modes

Figure 2-4 shows two transducers generating ultrasonic waves in the same piece. Note that the transducer on the left is producing longitudinal waves and that the transducer on the right is producing a different kind of wave. This different kind of wave is called a shear wave because the particle movement direction is at right angles to the wave movement direction. The velocity of shear waves through a material is approximately half that of the longitudinal waves. Note also that the transducer on the right is mounted on a plastic wedge so that the ultrasonic waves generated by the crystal enter the material at a specific angle. The specific angle required to produce only shear waves depends on the velocity of ultrasound within the material.

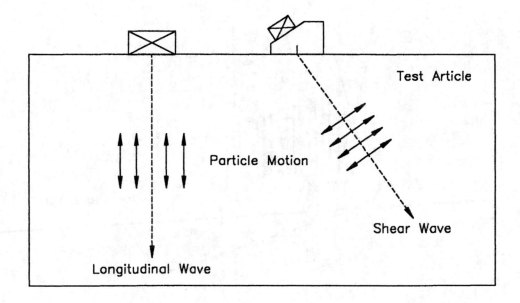

Figure 2-4. Longitudinal and Shear Wave Modes Compared

● Shear and Surface Waves

The particle displacements of shear waves are oriented in a plane normal to the direction of propagation. A special type of shear wave is confined to a thin layer of particles on the free boundary of a solid material. These waves are called surface or Rayleigh waves, and propagate with a velocity between 3 percent and 15 percent less than shear waves. As shown in Figure 2-5, when a transducer is mounted on a steeply-angled plastic wedge, the longitudinal beam in the wedge strikes the test surface at an angle resulting in a surface wave mode of sound travel in the test specimen. As shown, a surface wave can travel around a curve. Reflection of the surface wave occurs only at a sharp corner or at some discontinuity. The contact transducers that produce shear waves and surface waves are called angle beam transducers.

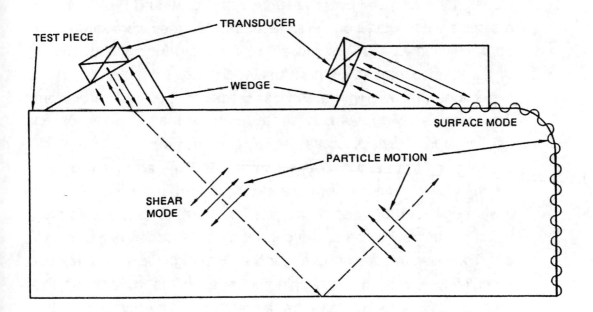

NOTE: The ultrasonic beams are longitudinal in each wedge. Mode conversion occurs when the ultrasound enters the test piece.

Figure 2-5. Shear and Surface Waves

- Transducer Beam Angles

Confusion may be encountered when angle beam transducers designed to produce a specific angle in one kind of material are applied to other materials with different acoustic velocities. A transducer designed to produce a shear wave beam at 45° in steel, for example, will produce a shear wave beam at 43° in aluminum or 30° in copper. Refer to "Refraction and Mode Conversion" later in this chapter.

- Rayleigh Waves

Rayleigh waves travel over the surface of a solid and bear a rough resemblance to waves on the surface of water; they were studied by Lord Rayleigh (c. 1875) because they are the principal component of disturbance from an earthquake at a distance from the epicenter. Reflections of Rayleigh waves from cracks in the surface or from discontinuities lying just beneath the surface may be seen on an oscilloscope. Rayleigh waves traveling on the top face of a block are reflected from a sharp edge corner, but if the edge is rounded off, the waves continue down the side face and are reflected at the lower edge and return to the origination point. These waves may travel the entire way around a cube if all of its edges are rounded off. They also travel around a cylinder. Rayleigh waves are almost completely absorbed by touching a finger to the surface, so the path of any reflection can be easily traced by observing the oscilloscope while moving the finger over the surface of the work. Rayleigh waves are also called surface waves, since their depth of penetration along the surface direction of travel is usually no more than one wavelength. The ultrasound travels along the surface with an elliptical particle motion as illustrated in Figure 2-6.

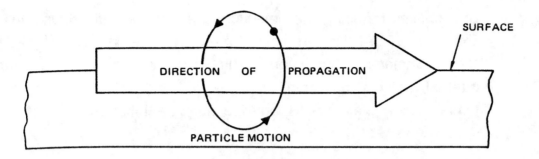

Figure 2-6. Rayleigh or Surface Waves

● Lamb Waves

If a surface wave is introduced into a material that has a thickness equal to three wavelengths or less of the beam, a different kind of wave results. The material begins to vibrate as a plate; i.e., the wave encompasses the entire thickness of the material. When this occurs, the normal rules for wave velocity along the plate break down. The velocity is no longer dependent upon the type of material and the type of wave. Instead, we get a wave velocity that is dependent on the frequency of the wave, the angle of incidence, and, of course, the type of material. The theory describing Lamb waves was developed by Horace Lamb (c. 1916), hence the name.

● Lamb Wave Types

There are two general types of Lamb (or plate) waves, depending on the way the particles in the material move as the wave moves along the plate. These are symmetrical and asymmetrical. Each type of Lamb wave has an infinite number of modes that the wave may attain. These modes are differentiated by the manner in which the particles in the material are moving. The ability of Lamb waves to propagate in thin plates makes them applicable to a wide variety of problems requiring the detection of subsurface discontinuities. Examples of practical problems for which plate waves are useful are: 1) immersion inspection of thin-walled tubing and plates for internal defects or grain size determinations; 2) testing for laminations in plate; and 3) changes in plate thickness.

Sound Beam Velocities

Ultrasonic waves travel through solids and liquids at relatively high speeds, but are more readily attenuated, or die out, in gases. The velocity of a specific mode of ultrasound is a constant through a given homogeneous material. The velocities of vibrational waves through various materials related to ultrasonic testing are listed by many authorities in centimeters per second x 100,000 (cm/s x 10^5) or inches per second x 100,000 (ips x 10^5). For convenience, velocities are given in this manual in centimeters per microsecond (cm/µs). Table 2-1 lists the velocities of a longitudinal wave through several different types of material to illustrate the wide range of velocities. These differences in velocity are due largely to differences in the density and elasticity of each material. Density alone cannot account for the extremely high velocity of sound in beryllium, which is less dense than aluminum. The acoustic velocity of water and mercury are almost identical, yet mercury is thirteen times as dense as water.

Table 2-1. Typical Ultrasonic Properties

MATERIAL	DENSITY (gm/cm³)	LONGITUDINAL WAVES	
		VELOCITY cm/µs	IMPEDANCE (gmx10³/cm²-s)
AIR	0.001	0.033	---
WATER	1.000	0.149	149
PLASTIC (ACRYLIC)	1.180	0.267	315
ALUMINUM (2117-T4)	2.800	0.625	1,750
BERYLLIUM	1.820	1.280	2,330
MERCURY	13.000	0.142	1,846

2-10

Acoustical Impedance

- General

  When a transducer is used to transmit an ultrasonic wave into a material, only part of the wave energy is transmitted; the rest is reflected at the interface between two different materials as ultrasound passes from one to the other. How much of the sound beam is reflected depends on a factor called the *acoustical impedance ratio*.

- Acoustical Impedance

  Acoustical impedance is a material property and can be generally referred to as the resistance of a material to the passage of sound waves. The specific acoustical impedance (Z) of any material may be computed by multiplying the density of the material (ρ) by the velocity of sound (V) through the material.

  $$Z = \rho V$$

  Air has a very low impedance while the impedance of water is relatively higher than the impedance of air. Aluminum and steel have still higher impedances.

- Impedance Ratio

  Impedance ratio between two materials is simply the acoustical impedance of one material divided by the acoustical impedance of the other material. When a sonic beam is passing from material one into material two, the impedance ratio is the impedance of the second material divided by the impedance of the first material. As the ratio increases, more of the original energy will be reflected.

Since air has a very small impedance, the impedance ratio between air and any liquid or solid material is very high. Therefore, most if not all of the ultrasound will be reflected at any interface between air and any other material.

An impedance ratio is often referred to as "an impedance mismatch." If the impedance ratio, for example, was 5/1, the impedance mismatch would be 5 to 1. The impedance ratio for a liquid-to-metal interface is on the order of 20 to 1 (approximately 80 percent reflection) while the impedance ratio for air-to-metal is about 100,000 to 1 (virtually 100 percent reflection). This results in only a small percentage of the ultrasonic energy transmitting into the test article. Ideally, a 1 to 1 impedance ratio would be desirable for the optimum transmission of ultrasound.

Ultrasound Reflection

In many ways, high-frequency vibrations act in the same way as light beams. For example, when they strike an Interrupting object, most of the energy is reflected. These reflections may then be picked up by a second or, in most cases, by the same crystal or transducer. Within the crystal the mechanical energy is transformed into electrical energy. The electrical energy is sent to the test system where it is amplified and presented. Ultrasonic testing does not give direct information about the exact nature of the discontinuity. This is deduced from several factors, the most important being a knowledge of the test piece material and its construction. Ultrasonic waves are reflected from both the discontinuity and the back surface of the test piece as indications which are also referred to as signals or echoes. The indication from the discontinuity is received before the back surface reflection is received. Figure 2-7 shows a situation where the time required for the ultrasound to travel through the test piece to the discontinuity and back is only two-thirds of the time required for the sound beam to reach to the back surface and return. This time differential indicates that the discontinuity is located two-thirds of the distance to the back surface.

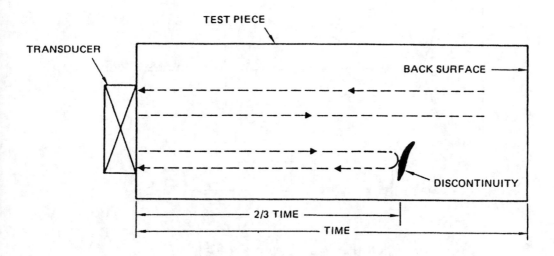

Figure 2-7. Sound Beam Reflection

Ultrasound Patterns

● General

In ultrasonic testing, the sound beam is generally considered to be a straight-sided projection of the face of the transducer. In reality, the beam is not all that consistent. If the beam intensity is measured at various distances from the transducer, two distinct zones are found as shown in Figure 2-8. These zones are known as the *near zone* (or Fresnel Zone) and the *far zone* or (Fraunhofer Zone).

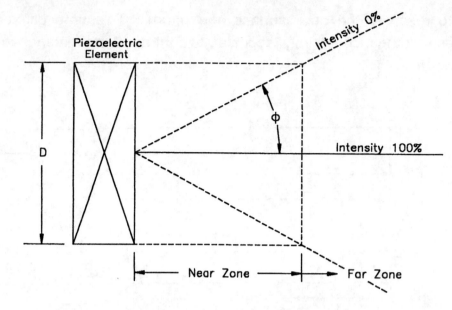

Figure 2-8. Beam Profile

●   Near Zone

In the zone closest to the transducer, the measurement of the ultrasonic intensities reveals an irregular pattern of localized high and low intensities.   This irregular pattern results from the interference between sound waves that are emitted from the face of the transducer.

The transducer may be considered to be a mosaic of crystals, or a plane source, each vibrating at the same frequency but slightly out of phase with each other.   Near the face of the crystal, the composite sound beam propagates chiefly as a plane-front wave; but spherical-front waves, which emanate from the periphery of the crystal face, produce side-lobe waves that interfere with the plane-front waves to cause patterns of acoustical maximums and minimums where they cross.

The effect that the presence of these acoustical patterns in the near zone will have on the ultrasonic test varies, but if the operator has proper knowledge of the presence of the near field, the proper test block can be scanned and those indications correlated with the indications obtained from the test.

The length of the near zone is dependent on the diameter of the transducer and the wavelength of the ultrasonic beam and may be computed from the equation:

$$N = \frac{D^2}{4\lambda}$$

where:

> N = length of the near zone
> D = transducer diameter
> λ = wavelength of the ultrasound

Since the wavelength of an ultrasonic beam in a particular material is inversely proportional to the frequency, the length of the near zone in a particular material can be shortened by lowering the frequency.

- Far Zone

In the region furthest from the transducer, the only effect of consequence is the spreading of the ultrasonic beam. Fraunhofer diffraction causes the beam to spread starting at the end of the near zone. At this distance, the beam appears to have originated at the center of the radiating face of the transducer and spread outward.

The degree of spread may be computed from the equation

$$\sin \phi = 1.22 \frac{\lambda}{D}$$

where:

ϕ = half-angle beam spread

λ = wavelength of the ultrasound

D = transducer diameter

Beam spread in steel, at various frequencies, is given in Figure 2-9. At any frequency, the larger the crystal, the narrower the beam; the smaller the crystal, the greater the beam spread. At any diameter, higher frequencies result in narrower beam spread than lower frequencies. The diameter of the transducer is often limited by the size of the available contact surface. Transducers smaller than 1/8-inch (3.2 mm) diameter have been used. For shallow depth testing, 3/8 inch diameter (9.5 mm) and 1/2 inch diameter (12.7 mm) transducers are used at the higher frequencies such as 5.0 to 25.0 MHz. The large-diameter transducer is usually selected for testing through greater depths of material due to its increased power.

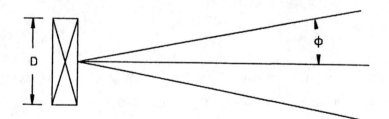

FREQUENCY MHz	λ in.	TRANSDUCER DIAMETER (D) INCHES			
		3/8	1/2	3/4	1.0
1.0	0.230	48°	34°	22°	16°
2.25	0.102	19°	14°	10°	7°
5.0	0.046	9°	6°	4°	3°

Figure 2-9. Beam Spread in Steel

Figure 2-10 shows the reduction in beam spread in steel for a 1/2-inch-diameter (12.7 mm) transducer when the frequency is raised from 1.0 MHz to 2.25 MHz. The secondary or side lobes shown in the figure are edge effects caused by the manner of crystal mounting. In practical work, the primary beam is the only one of consequence. Secondary beams are considered when the geometry of the test specimen is such that the secondary beams are reflected back to the transducer, creating spurious effects. The strongest intensity of the sound beam is along its central axis with a gradual reduction in amplitude away from the axis.

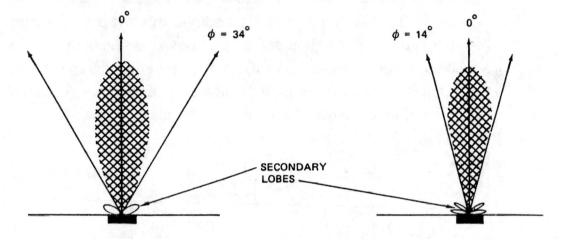

f = 1.0 MHz
λ = 0.230 in. (5.8 mm)
D = 0.5 in. (12.7 mm)

f = 2.25 MHz
λ = 0.102 in. (2.6 mm)
D = 0.5 in. (12.7 mm)

Figure 2-10. Sound Beam Radiation Patterns

Refraction and Mode Conversion

- General

  Refraction and mode conversion of the ultrasonic beam as it passes at an angle from one material to another are comparable to the refraction of light beams when passing from one medium to another. The angles given are based on typical ultrasonic velocities for these mediums and are approximate.

  Figure 2-11 shows a transducer inducing a longitudinal sound beam into water. The water transmits the beam to the test piece. When the longitudinal wave (L-wave) sound beam is incident to the surface of the test specimen in the normal (perpendicular) direction, the beam is transmitted through the first and second medium as a 100 percent longitudinal beam and no refraction occurs.

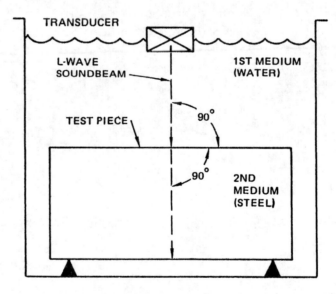

Figure 2-11. Normal Incident Beam

- **Mixed Mode Conversion**

As shown in Figure 2-12, as the incident angle is changed from the initial 90° position, refraction and mode conversion occur and the original longitudinal beam is transmitted into the second medium as varying percentages of both longitudinal and shear wave beams. As illustrated for water and steel, the refracted angle for the L-wave beam is four times the incident angle, and the S-wave beam angle is a little more than twice the incident angle. If the incident angle is rotated further, the refraction angles of the L-wave and the S-wave increase.

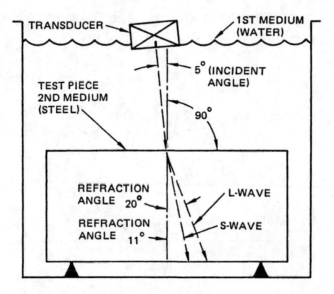

Figure 2-12. 5° Incident Beam

Refraction and mode conversion occur because the L-wave velocity changes when the beam enters the second medium. The velocity of the shear wave is approximately half that of the longitudinal wave. As the incident angle is rotated further, both refracted angles increase. The first beam to reach a refraction angle of 90° will be the L-wave.

- Shear Wave Generation

When the transducer is rotated to an incident angle of approximately 15°, the refracted angle of the L-wave is increased to 90° and the L-wave is totally reflected from the test surface as shown in Figure 2-13. This incident angle is called the First Critical Angle (the angle where the L-wave beam is totally reflected and only S-wave beams are transmitted through the second medium).

Further rotation of the transducer increases the angle of the refracted shear wave beam. When the S-wave beam reaches 90°, the resultant incident angle is termed the Second Critical Angle. In the entire region between the First and Second Critical Angle, only S-wave beams are produced.

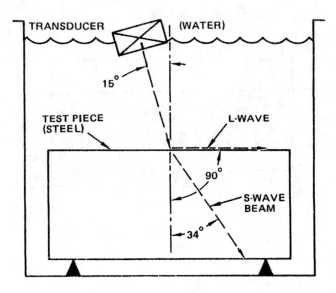

Figure 2-13. First Critical Angle

- Surface Wave Generation

When the transducer is rotated to an incident angle of about 27°, the S-wave refraction angle is increased to 90°. Figure 2-14 shows that the only reflected waves are L-waves. At slightly (approximately 5°) increased angles of incidence a surface wave is generated. The surface wave has some particle disturbance in the test surface; however, these waves are rapidly attenuated by the water medium. The shear waves are not reflected because they do not propagate in a liquid or gaseous medium.

In contact testing, where the transducer is placed directly on the test piece, surface waves are produced at angles just beyond the Second Critical Angle. Surface waves serve a function in ultrasonic testing and their presence can be readily detected.

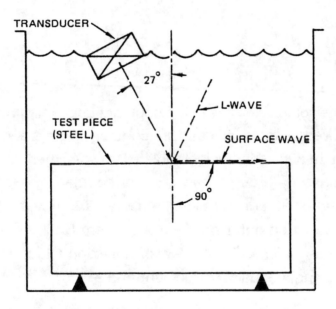

Figure 2-14. Second Critical Angle

- Summary

To summarize, the critical angles are the incident angles at which either the longitudinal or shear wave travels along the surface of the second medium. For those incident angles beyond the Second Critical Angle there is total reflection of the beam, and no ultrasound energy is transmitted into the second medium.

In contact testing, the incident angle slightly beyond the Second Critical Angle produces surface waves in the test specimen.

Both critical angles may be calculated by an equation derived from Snell's Law if the velocities of the sound beam in the first and second medium are known or can be established.

Snell's Law

- General

When the sonic velocities in the couplant used in immersion testing or the wedge material used in contact angle beam testing are different than the sonic velocity in the test specimen, the longitudinal waves passing through the wedge or couplant are refracted when the sound beam enters the test material. Refracted angles may be computed by an equation developed from Snell's Law. Reflected waves are governed by the law of reflection which states that the reflected angle equals the incident angle.

- Snell's Law Calculations

  Snell's Law states that the ratio of the sine of the angle of incidence to the sine of the angle of refraction equals the ratio of the corresponding wave velocities.

  Snell's Law can be expressed mathematically as follows:

  $$\frac{\sin \phi_I}{\sin \phi_R} = \frac{V_I}{V_R}$$

  Where:

  > ϕ_I = incident angle from normal in the liquid or wedge
  > ϕ_R = angle of the refracted beam in the test material
  > V_I = velocity of incident beam in the liquid or wedge
  > V_R = velocity of refracted beam in the test material

  NOTE: The calculations for determining angles of incidence or refraction require the use of trigonometric tables (Appendix D). The sine (abbr: sin) ratios are given In decimal fractions. Velocities are given in centimeters per microsecond (cm/µs) in Appendix E. To convert cm/µs to cm/s x 10^5, move the decimal one place to the right. Divide cm/µs by 2.54 to obtain in/µs.

- Typical Problem Solving Method

  Figure 2-15 shows a contact transducer mounted at an incident angle of 35° on a plastic wedge. The angle of the refracted beam may be calculated with Snell's Law since the incident angle and the velocity of the sound beam in the first and second medium are known. In this case, only shear waves are produced in the steel, as the incident angle is in the region between the First and Second Critical Angles.

Problem: Calculate the angle of refraction for longitudinal waves and shear waves as they enter a steel specimen from a plastic wedge at an incident angle of 35° as illustrated in the following test set-up.

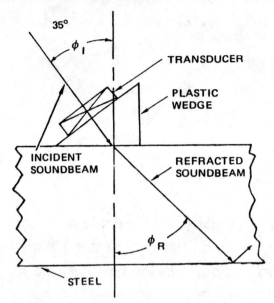

$$\frac{\sin \phi_I}{\sin \phi_R} = \frac{V_I}{V_R}$$

Given:

$V_I = 0.267$ cm/µs

$V_R = 0.585$ cm/µs (L-waves in steel)

$V_R = 0.323$ cm/µs (S-waves in steel)

$\sin \phi_I = \sin 35° = 0.574$

Solution for L-waves

By substitution into Snell's Law we have:

$$\frac{\sin 35°}{\sin \phi_R} = \frac{0.267}{0.585}$$

$$\sin \phi_R = \frac{0.585\ (0.574)}{0.267}$$

$$\sin \phi_R = 1.258$$

Because the $\sin^{-1}$ of 1.258 is undefined, all L-waves are reflected.

Solution for S-waves

By substitution into Snell's Law we have:

$$\frac{\sin 35°}{\sin \phi_R} = \frac{0.267}{0.323}$$

$$\sin \phi_R = \frac{0.323\ (0.574)}{0.267}$$

$$\sin \phi_R = 0.694$$

$$\phi_R = 44°$$

S-waves are refracted at an angle of 44°.

Figure 2-15. Application of Snell's Law for the
Calculation of Refracted Angles

Critical Angles of Refraction

- General

Sound beams passing through a medium such as water or plastic are refracted when entering a second medium at an incident angle. For small incident beam angles, sound beams are refracted and subjected to mode conversion resulting in a combination of shear and longitudinal waves. The region between normal incidence and the First Critical Angle is not used as commonly for ultrasonic testing as is the region beyond the First Critical Angle where only shear waves are produced. The presence of both the longitudinal and shear waves creates additional display interpretation difficulties for the ultrasonic operator.

- First Critical Angle

As the angle of incidence is increased, the First Critical Angle is reached when the refracted longitudinal beam angle reaches 90°. At this point, only shear waves exist in the second medium. When selecting a contact shear wave angle beam transducer, or when adjusting an immersed transducer at an incident angle to produce shear waves, two conditions are considered. First, and of prime importance, is that the refracted longitudinal wave must be totally reflected (its angle of refraction must be 90° or greater) so that the penetrating beam is limited to shear waves only. Second, within the limits of the first condition, the refracted shear wave must enter the test piece in accordance with the requirements of the test procedure. In immersion testing, the First Critical Angle is calculated to make certain that the probe is positioned so that the sound beam enters the test material at the desired angle in the area of interest.

● Calculation of Critical Angles

If the sound beam velocities for the incident wave and for the refracted wave are known (V_I and V_R), either critical angle may be calculated with the formula for Snell's Law using the sine of 90° (which is 1) as the sine of the refracted angle in the second medium. Thus, to compute the First Critical Angle in the case of the contact transducer mounted on a plastic wedge for testing steel:

$$Snell's\ Law: \quad \frac{\sin \phi_I}{\sin \phi_R} = \frac{V_I}{V_R\ (longitudinal\ wave)}$$

$$\frac{\sin \phi_I}{\sin \phi_R\ (1.00)} = \frac{0.267\ cm/\mu s}{0.585\ cm/\mu s}$$

Divide V_R into V_I = 0.456 = 27° for First Critical Angle. If the Second Critical Angle is desired, V_R is the sound beam velocity for a shear wave in steel: 0.323 cm/µs. V_R is again divided into V_I = 0.827 = 56° for the Second Critical Angle.

- Table 2-2 lists approximate critical angles for various test materials when water is used as the first medium (V_I = 0.149 cm/µs).

- Table 2-3 lists approximate critical angles for the same test materials when a plastic wedge is used as the first medium (V_I = 0.267 cm/µs). Note that uranium does not have a second critical angle in this case. This is because the shear wave velocity in uranium is less than the longitudinal wave velocity in plastic. Essentially this means that the incident angle would have to be greater than 90° to obtain a 90° refraction of the beam in uranium.

Table 2-2. Critical Angles, Immersion Testing

First Medium is H_2O (V = 0.149 cm/μs)

TEST MATERIAL	1ST CRITICAL ANGLE	2ND CRITICAL ANGLE	VELOCITY (cm/μs)	
			LONGITUDINAL	SHEAR
BERYLLIUM	7°	10°	1.280	0.871
ALUMINUM, 2117-T4	14°	29°	0.625	0.310
STEEL	15°	27°	0.585	0.323
STAINLESS, 302	15°	29°	0.566	0.312
TUNGSTEN	17°	31°	0.518	0.287
URANIUM	26°	51°	0.338	0.193

Table 2-3. Critical Angles, Contact Testing

First Medium is Plastic (V = 0.267 cm/μs)

TEST MATERIAL	1ST CRITICAL ANGLE	2ND CRITICAL ANGLE	VELOCITY (cm/μs)	
			LONGITUDINAL	SHEAR
BERYLLIUM	12°	18°	1.280	0.871
ALUMINUM, 2117-T4	25°	59°	0.625	0.310
STEEL	27°	56°	0.585	0.323
STAINLESS, 302	28°	59°	0.566	0.312
TUNGSTEN	31°	68°	0.518	0.287
URANIUM	52°	-	0.338	0.193

CONTACT TESTING

● General

Contact testing is divided into three techniques which are determined by the sound beam wave mode desired: the straight beam technique for transmitting longitudinal waves in the test specimen, the angle beam technique for generating shear waves, and the angle beam surface wave technique for producing Rayleigh or Lamb waves. Transducers used in these techniques are held in direct contact with the material using a thin liquid film for a couplant. The couplant selected should be high enough in viscosity to remain on the test surface during the test. For most contact testing, the couplant should be relatively thin and should be selected to provide the proper impedance match.

- Straight Beam Techniques

The straight beam technique is accomplished by projecting a sound beam perpendicularly to the test surface on the test specimen to obtain pulse-echo reflections from the back surface or from discontinuities which lie between the two surfaces. To avoid confusion from dead zone and near zone effects encountered with straight beam transducers, parts with a thickness less than 5/8 inch (15.9 mm) are tested with straight beam probes that utilize a delay line or stand-off to absorb these effects. This technique is also used in the through-transmission technique using two transducers where the internal discontinuities interrupt the sound beam causing a reduction in the received signal.

   - Pulse-Echo Techniques

Pulse-echo techniques may use either single or double straight beam transducers. Figure 2-16 shows the single-unit straight beam transducer in use. With the single unit, the transducer acts as both transmitter and receiver projecting a pulsed beam of longitudinal waves into the specimen and receiving reflections from the back surface and from any discontinuity lying in the beam path. The double transducer or dual-element transducer unit is useful when the test surface is rough or when the specimen shape is irregular and the back surface is not parallel with the front surface. One transducer transmits and the other receives as shown in

Figure 2-17. In this case, the receiver will receive discontinuity reflections and may receive back surface reflections.

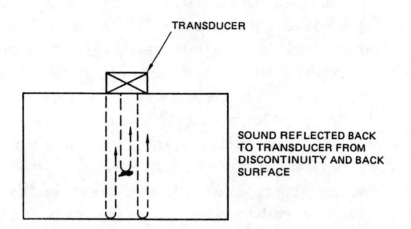

TRANSDUCER

SOUND REFLECTED BACK
TO TRANSDUCER FROM
DISCONTINUITY AND BACK
SURFACE

Figure 2-16. Single Transducer Pulse-Echo Technique

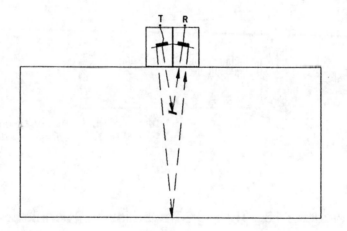

Figure 2-17. Dual-Element Transducer Pulse-Echo Technique

— Through-Transmission Techniques

Two transducers are used in the through-transmission technique—one on each side of the test specimen as shown in Figure 2-18. One unit acts as a transmitter and the other as a receiver. The transmitter unit projects a sound beam into the material. The beam travels through the material to the opposite surface, and the sound is picked up at the opposite surface by the receiving unit. Any discontinuities in the path of the sound beam cause a reduction in the amount of sound energy reaching the receiving unit. For best results in this technique, the transmitter utilizes a crystal that is the best available generator of acoustic energy, and the receiver utilizes a crystal that is the best available receiver of acoustic energy.

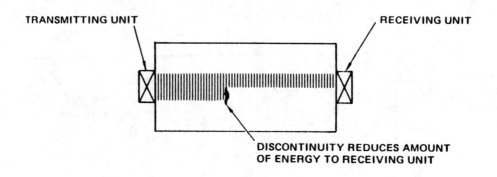

Figure 2-18. Through-Transmission Technique

● Angle Beam Techniques

The angle beam technique is used to transmit sound waves into the test material at a predetermined angle to the test surface. According to the angle selected, the wave modes produced in the test material may be mixed longitudinal and shear (bimodal), shear only, or surface modes. Usually shear wave transducers are used in angle beam testing. Figure 2-19 shows an angle beam unit scanning plate and pipe material. In the angle beam technique, the sound beam enters the test material at an angle and proceeds by successive zig-zag reflections from the specimen boundaries until it is interrupted by a discontinuity or an acoustical interface oriented perpendicular to it where it reverses direction and is reflected back to the transducer. Angle beam techniques are used for testing welds, pipe or tubing, sheet and plate material, and for specimens of irregular shape where straight beam units are unable to contact all of the surface. Angle beam transducers are identified by case markings that show the refracted angle (usually in steel) though no standard exists for marking probes.

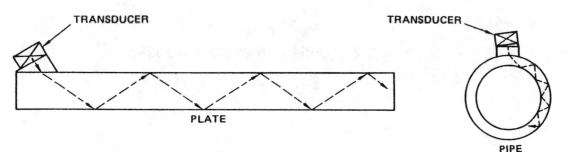

Figure 2-19. Angle Beam Technique

- Surface Wave Techniques

  The surface wave technique requires special angle beam transducers that project the sound beam into the test specimen at an angle slightly beyond the second critical angle. For test specimens where near-surface discontinuities are encountered, surface wave transducers are used to generate Rayleigh surface waves in the test material. The surface wave technique is shown in Figure 2-20.

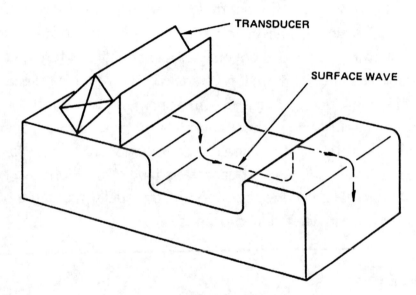

Figure 2-20. Surface Wave Technique

Immersion Testing

- General

  Any one of the following three techniques may be used in the immersion method.

- The immersion technique where both the transducer and the test specimen are immersed in water

- The bubbler or squirter technique where the sound beam is transmitted through a column of flowing water

- The wheel transducer technique, where the transducer is mounted in the axle of a liquid-filled tire that rolls on the test surface

The sound beam is directed through the water into the material using either a straight beam technique for generating longitudinal waves or one of the many angle beam techniques for generating shear waves.

Ultrasonic Displays

- General

There are three common types of displays utilized with ultrasonic tests. These are the A-scan, B-scan and C-scan displays. The A-scan display presents time or distance horizontally and reflected sound (or amplitude) vertically. The B-scan represents an end or cross-sectional view of the specimen and the C-scan represents a plan (or top) view of the specimen. Other data display methods are available such as D-scan and P-scan which are somewhat specialized and will not be further discussed. Computerized equipment makes possible the simultaneous data collection and color-coded display of all three representations.

Influence of the Test Specimen on the Sound Beam

- General

  The highest degree of reliability in ultrasonic testing is obtained when the influence of test specimen variables and their effects are understood and considered. A shortcut for evaluating the effects of test specimen geometry and material properties is to drill flat-bottomed holes, or other suitable reflectors, in one of the test parts and then to use that part as a reference standard. With or without such a standard, the operator must be familiar with the influence of geometric and material variables. In one form or another, the operator will receive spurious or confusing indications from any of the following test specimen variables.

  - Surface Roughness

    Rough surfaces distort ultrasonic indications as follows:

    - Loss of echo amplitude from discontinuities within the part. This loss may be due to scatter at the surface of the part or to roughness of the surface on the discontinuity.

    - Loss of resolving power (the ability to distinguish between two closely spaced reflectors) which is caused by a widening of the initial pulse (the initial electrical pulse from the instruments pulser circuit) caused by reflection of transducer side- or secondary-lobe energy. Side-lobe energy is normally not reflected back into the transducer from smooth surfaces. This condition may mask the presence of a discontinuity just below the surface.

- Widening of the ultrasonic beam due to scatter caused by the rough surface or due to a requirement for a lower frequency to reduce scatter.

— Shape or Contour of Specimen

Angular (nonparallel) boundaries or contoured surfaces of the test specimen cause partial or total loss of reflection. Figure 2-21 shows a test specimen with an irregular back surface. In the area where the back surface is parallel to the front surface, the sound waves are returned to the transducer. On the left side, in the area where the back surface is sloped at an angle from the front surface, the sound waves are reflected from one boundary to another until they die out from attenuation. In actual practice, portions of the sound beam are spread from each reflection point so that a few weak signals may be received by the transducer. These signals create confusing indications.

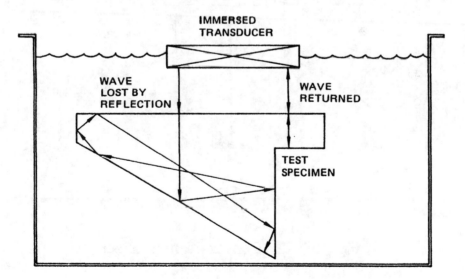

Figure 2-21. Irregular Back Surface Effect

- A convex surface on the test specimen is shown in Figure 2-22. The sound beam is widened by refraction after passing through the convex boundary. Considerable ultrasonic energy is lost by reflection at the test specimen surface as shown, and by beam spread. Signals reflected from the discontinuity have less amplitude than signals received from a discontinuity of the same size in a flat test specimen.

- Figure 2-23 shows a test specimen with a concave surface. After passing through the concave boundary, the sound beam is narrowed or focused. The discontinuity signals are relatively high in amplitude but may be difficult to identify because of unwanted reflections from the test surface.

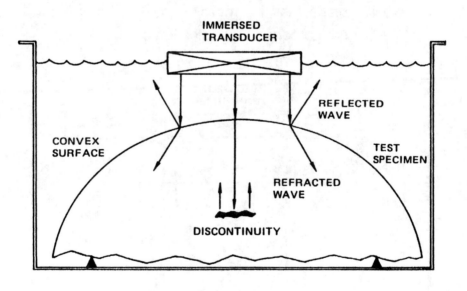

Figure 2-22. Convex Surface Effect

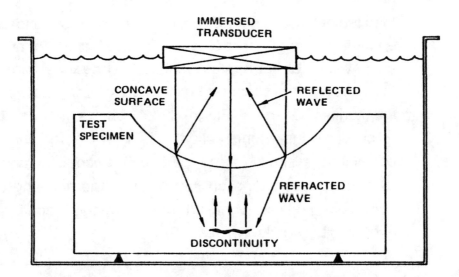

Figure 2-23. Concave Surface Effect

– Mode Conversion Within Test Specimen

When the shape or contour of the test specimen is such that the sound beam, or a portion of it as in the case of beam spread, is not reflected directly back to the transducer, mode conversion occurs at the boundary points contacted by the beam. If a direct reflection is obtained, mode conversion indications may be identified as they will appear behind the first reflection. These echoes are slow to appear because they are slowed by velocity changes when they are changed from longitudinal waves to shear waves and then back to longitudinal waves during mode conversion. Sound beams are reflected at angles which are governed by the law of reflection. Snell's Law can be used to calculate the refracted and reflected angles.

As the incident angle of the longitudinal beam is known or can be easily determined, the angle of the reflected longitudinal beam is known, since the angle of incidence is equal to the angle of reflection. The reflected shear beam angle will be about half the longitudinal beam angle, since the velocity of the shear beam is about half the velocity of the longitudinal beam. Figure 2-24 shows sound beam reflections within a long, solid test part. The spreading beam contacts the sides of the part with a specific angle of incidence. Depending on the material, the resulting mode conversion consists of mixed modes of longitudinal, shear, and possibly surface waves.

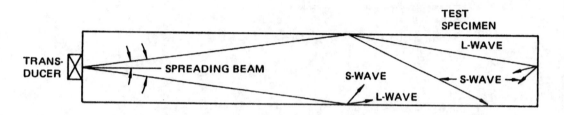

Figure 2-24. Mode Conversion Caused by Beam Spread

- Coarse Grains Within Test Specimen

  Coarse or large grains within the test specimen can cause scatter and loss of reflections or multiple nonrelevant indications, particularly when the size of the grain and the wavelength are comparable. If the frequency is lowered to the point where the wavelength is greater than the grain size, scattering losses are reduced but sensitivity is lowered.

- Orientation and Depth of Discontinuity

  The orientation and depth of the discontinuity may cause confusing indications, or may result in the loss of the discontinuity echo. In the case of orientation, the discontinuity may lie with its long axis parallel to the sound beam causing a small indication in proportion to the size of the discontinuity. If the discontinuity is angled from the sound beam, its reflections are directed away from the transducer. A sudden loss of a back surface reflection while scanning can indicate the presence of such a discontinuity. If the decrease in amplitude of the back surface deflection is proportional to the indication caused by the reflection from the discontinuity, the discontinuity is flat and parallel to the test surface. If the discontinuity indication is small compared to the loss of back surface reflection, the discontinuity is probably at an angle other than parallel to the test surface.

The extent of the near zone is determined by the formula presented earlier (page 2-15). Sound beam intensity is irregular in the near zone, causing a condition where varying indications may be obtained from the same discontinuity as the transducer is moved across it.

Beyond the near zone in the far zone, the amplitude of the indication from the discontinuity diminishes exponentially as the distance increases.

Reference Table

Appendix E lists the acoustic properties of several materials. Included in the table are the density of each material and the velocity and impedance of longitudinal, shear, and surface waves in each material. Density is given in grams per cubic centimeter (gm/cm^3) while the wave velocity is given in centimeters per microsecond (cm/μs) and the impedance is given in grams times 10^3 per square centimeter-second (gm x 10^3/cm^2-s).

CHAPTER 3: EQUIPMENT

TABLE OF CONTENTS

TABLE OF CONTENTS (CONT'D.)

LIST OF FIGURES

LIST OF FIGURES (CONT'D.)

LIST OF TABLES

Table   Page

CHAPTER 3

EQUIPMENT

Piezoelectricity

To produce an ultrasonic beam in a test piece, a transmitter applies high-frequency electrical pulses to a "piezoelectric" crystal. The prefix "piezo" is derived from a Greek word meaning "to press." The first two syllables should be pronounced like the words "pie" and "ease." Piezoelectricity refers to a reversible phenomenon whereby a crystal, when vibrated, produces an electric current or, conversely, when an electric current is applied to the crystal it vibrates. When energized with electrical pulses the crystal transforms the electrical energy into mechanical vibrations and transmits the vibrations through a coupling medium, such as water or oil, into the test material. These pulsed vibrations propagate through the object with a velocity that depends on the density and elasticity of the test material.

Sound Beam Frequencies

Most ultrasonic search units have frequencies available in a range from 0.5 MHz to 25 MHz. These vibrations, which are far beyond the audible range for humans, propagate in the test material as waves of particle vibrations. Ultrasound of all frequencies can penetrate fine-grained material without difficulty. However, when using high frequencies in coarse-grained material, interference in the form of scattering may be expected. Greater depth of penetration may be achieved by using lower frequencies. Selection of the test frequency is governed by the nature of the particular problem. Ultrasound with low frequencies (up to about 1 MHz) readily penetrate through most materials because of the small amount of attenuation of low frequencies. They are also scattered less by a coarse grain structure and can be used when the test surface is rough. On the debit side, the angle of divergence of low-frequency beams is large, making it difficult to resolve small flaws. High-frequency transducers emit a more concentrated beam with better resolving power. Limitations in the use of high frequencies are the extended near zone and the increased scattering by coarse-grained metals. All available frequencies may be used in immersion testing. The extended near zone is the main reason higher frequencies (above 10 MHz) are not generally used in contact testing. As the frequency of ultrasonic vibrations increases, the wavelength correspondingly decreases and approaches the dimensions of the grains in a metal.

Sound Beam Attenuation

High-frequency ultrasound passing through a material is reduced in power or attenuated by reflection and scattering of the beams at the grain boundaries. This loss is proportional to the grain size in the material and the wavelength of the beam. Scattering losses are greatest where the wavelength is less than one-third the grain size. As the frequency is lowered and the wavelength becomes greater than the grain size, attenuation is due primarily to absorption of the wave. Wave energy is lost through heat due to friction of the vibrating particles.

Time/Distance Relationship

The round trip distance that the sound beam travels to a reflecting surface can be measured on the cathode-ray tube (CRT) as illustrated in Figure 3-1. The initial pulse, or main bang, and the echo (sound beam traveling through water in this illustration) from the reflecting surface produce two sharp indications on the baseline. The indication at the left (A) results from the initial pulse while the indication at the right (B) is the indication from the front surface of the plate under test. The distance between the two indications is proportional to the distance between the transducer and the front surface of the specimen.

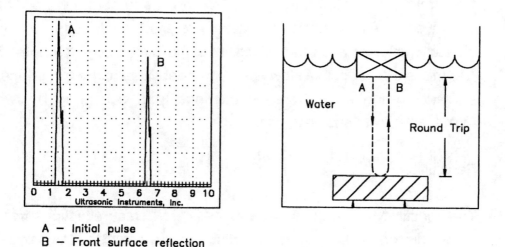

A — Initial pulse
B — Front surface reflection

Figure 3-1. Time/Distance Measuring

As mentioned earlier, time and distance measurements are related. In later discussion, it will be seen that the baseline may be adjusted to match the number of screen divisions involved in the round trip distance (as illustrated).

Transducers

- **General**

  In ultrasonic testing, the "eye" and "ear" of the system is the transducer. After transmitting the ultrasound energy, the transducer receives reflections that result from the condition of the material. It then relays the information back to the instrument where it is displayed. As is often the case, detailed evaluation of the characteristics of each transducer may be necessary. Chapter 5 describes that process. However, the capabilities of the transducer and the testing system are for the most part described by two terms: sensitivity and resolution.

- **Sensitivity**

  The sensitivity of a transducer is its ability to detect reflections from small discontinuities at given distances. Precise transducer sensitivity is unique to a specific transducer. Even transducers manufactured by the same company of the same size, frequency, and material do not always produce identical indications. Transducer sensitivity is the ability to detect and process the reflected energy from a given size discontinuity at a specific sound-path distance in a reference block.

- **Resolution**

  The resolution, or resolving power, of a transducer refers to its ability to separate indications from two targets close together in position or depth (for example, the front surface indication and the indication from a small discontinuity just beneath the surface). The time required for the transducer to stop "ringing" or vibrating after having been supplied with a large voltage pulse is a measure of its resolving power. Long "tails" or transmissions of sound energy from a ringing transducer cause a wide, high-amplitude front surface indication. In this case, a small discontinuity just beneath the surface is masked by the ringing signal.

- Materials

Developments in man-made polarized ceramics have produced the most efficient crystals for applying ultrasonic energy. They operate on low voltage, are practically unaffected by moisture, and are usable at high temperatures up to 1112°F (600°C). They are limited, however, by their relatively low mechanical strength, some mode conversion interference, and a tendency to age (i.e., to lose their polarization and become very brittle).

The most commonly used piezoceramics include sodium bismuth titanate, lead metaniobate, lead titanate and several variations within the lead zirconate titanate (PZT) family. These include PZT4, PZT5H, PZT7A and PZT8. These PZT materials are selected for applications dependent upon their specific characteristics. Additionally, PZT comes in the form of a composite.

Table 3-1 describes a few characteristics of these crystals. It is not important that you remember the details but rather that you understand that piezoceramics offer a tremendous array of possibilities.

Table 3-1. Characteristics of Common Piezoelectric Materials

Crystal Material	Characteristics/Applications
Lead Metaniobate #1	Good power; great receiver; broad band; high temperature applications
Lead Metaniobate #2	Good transmitter and receiver; narrow band; contact transducers ≥2 MHz
PZT4	Good transmitter and receiver; best at lower frequencies; good penetrator of coarse-grained materials; high power applications
PZT5H	Great penetrator; good receiver; multifrequency; accelerometers
Lead Titanate	Great receiver; good penetrator; good at higher frequencies; medical diagnostics
Sodium Bismuth Titanate	Extremely stable; ultrahigh temperature applications

● Transducer Types

Transducers are made in a limitless number of sizes and shapes from extremely small (pinpoint) to 6-inch-wide (15.2 cm) "paintbrush" transducers. The many shapes are the result of much experience and the requirement for many special applications. Size of a transducer is a contributing factor to its performance. For instance, the larger the transducer, the narrower the sound beam (less beam spread) for a given frequency. The narrower beams of the larger (beyond 1 inch or 25.4 mm) high-frequency transducers have greater ability for detecting very small discontinuities. The larger transducers also transmit more energy into the test part, so they can be used to gain deep penetration. The large, single-crystal transducers are generally limited to lower frequencies (≤5 MHz) because the very thin high-frequency crystals are fragile.

- Contact Transducers

  Contact transducers are made for both straight and angle beam testing. When the straight beam unit is faced with a wear plate, an electrode on the front face of the crystal provides for an internal ground. All angle beam and immersion-type transducers are internally grounded. In addition, the immersion-type transducers, including the coaxial cable connection, are waterproof since, in use, they are completely submerged.

- Angle Beam Transducers

  Transducers are also classified as either straight beam transducers or angle beam transducers. The term "straight beam" means that the energy from the transducer is transmitted into the test specimen in a direction normal (perpendicular) to the test surface. Angle beam transducers direct the sound beam into the test specimen surface at an angle other than 90°. Angle beam transducers are used to locate discontinuities oriented at angles to the surface and to determine the size of discontinuities oriented at angles other than parallel to the surface. Angled transducers are also used to propagate shear, surface, and plate waves into the test specimen by mode conversion. In contact testing, angle beam transducers use a wedge, usually of plastic (Lucite), between the transducer face and the surface of the test specimen to direct the ultrasound into the test surface at the desired angle. In immersion testing, angulation of the beam is accomplished by varying the angle of a straight beam transducer to direct the beam into the test part at the desired angle. Both straight and angled transducers are shown in Figure 3-2.

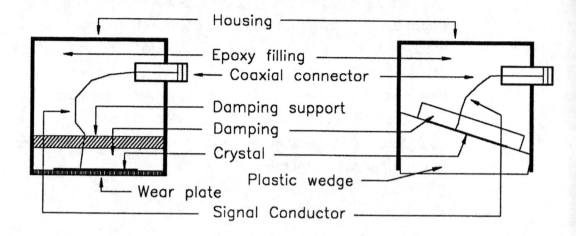

Housing

Epoxy filling

Coaxial connector

Damping support

Damping

Crystal

Plastic wedge

Wear plate

Signal Conductor

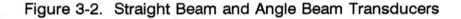

Figure 3-2. Straight Beam and Angle Beam Transducers

− Dual-Element (Double) Transducers

The dual-element transducer differs from the single transducer in that, while the single transducer may be a transmitter only, a receiver only, or both transmitter and receiver, the dual-element probe is in essence two single transducers mounted in the same housing for pitch-and-catch testing. In the dual-element (dual) search unit, one transducer is the transmitter and the other is the receiver. They may be mounted side by side for straight beam testing and mounted stacked or tandem for angle beam testing. In all cases, the crystals are separated by a sound barrier to block cross-talk. Figure 3-3 shows both types of dual-element transducers.

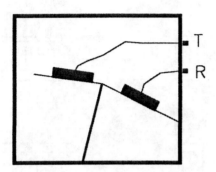

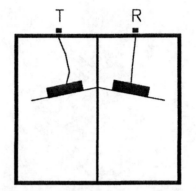

Tandem Angle Beam

Paired Crystals

Figure 3-3. Typical Dual-Element Transducers

— Paintbrush Transducers

The wide (6 inch or 15.2 cm) paintbrush transducers are made up of a mosaic pattern of smaller crystals carefully matched so that the intensity of the beam pattern varies very little over the entire length of the transducer. This is necessary to maintain uniform sensitivity. Paintbrush transducers provide a long, narrow, rectangular beam (in cross section) for scanning large surfaces. Their purpose is to quickly discover discontinuities in the test specimen.

Smaller, more sensitive transducers are then used to define the size, shape, orientation, and exact location of the discontinuities. Figure 3-4 shows a typical paintbrush transducer.

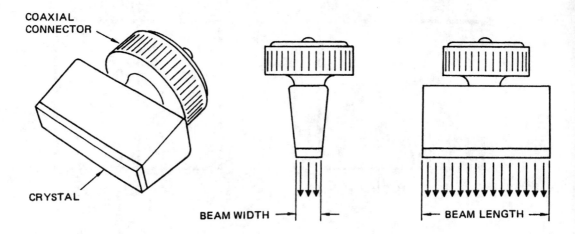

Figure 3-4. Typical Paintbrush Transducer

— Faced Unit or Contour Focused Transducers

In addition to wedges, other frontal members are added to the transducer for various reasons. On contact transducers, wear plates are often added to protect the fragile crystal from wear, breakage, or the harmful effects of foreign substances and to protect the front electrode. Frontal units shaped to direct the ultrasound perpendicular to the surface at all points on curved surfaces and radii are known as contour-correction lenses. These lenses sharpen the front surface indication by equalizing the sound-path distance between the transducer and the test surface. A comparison of flat and contoured transducers is shown in Figure 3-5.

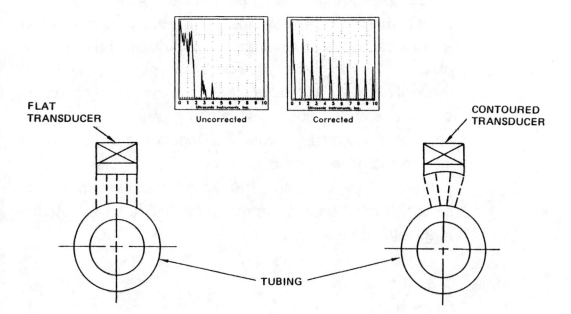

FLAT
TRANSDUCER

Uncorrected

Corrected

CONTOURED
TRANSDUCER

TUBING

Figure 3-5. Flat and Contour-Corrected Transducers

Other acoustic lenses focus the sound beam from the transducer much as light beams are focused. Cylindrically focused transducers concentrate the ultrasound into a long, narrow, blunt-pointed beam of increased intensity which is capable of detecting very small discontinuities in a relatively small area. Spherically focused transducers focus the sound beam to a point within a test article. Focusing the sound beam moves its point of maximum intensity towards the transducer, but shortens its usable range. The test specimen has the effect of a second lens in this case.

When the beam enters the test surface it is refracted, as shown in Figure 3-6. The increased intensity produces increased sensitivity at and near the focal point. Moving the point of maximum intensity closer to the transducer (which is also closer to the test surface) improves the near surface resolution. The disturbing effects of rough surface and material noise are also reduced. This is true simply because a smaller cross-sectional area is being tested. In a smaller cross-sectional area, the true discontinuity indications will be relatively large compared to the combined noise of other nonrelevant indications. The useful thickness range of focused transducers is approximately 0.010 to 2.0 inches (0.25 to 50.8 mm).

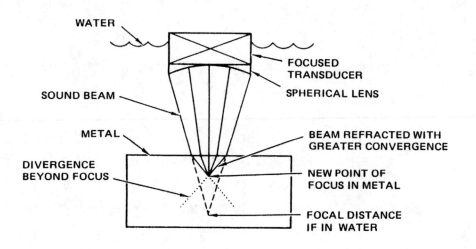

Figure 3-6. A Focused Beam in Metal

- Electronically-Focused Transducers

    Special transducers, known as "linear arrays," can be focused
    using electronic phase control. A typical linear array is
    shown in Figure 3-7. The linear array is a collection of very
    small transducers with each transducer able to act as a
    transmitter or receiver. Transducer width may be as small as
    0.020 inches (0.5 mm) and an array may consist of several
    hundred small transducers. By selectively pulsing each
    transducer or group of transducers in a given order, the
    ultrasonic beam may be focused in sound path or may cause
    the focused beam to sweep across the test specimen without
    moving the array.

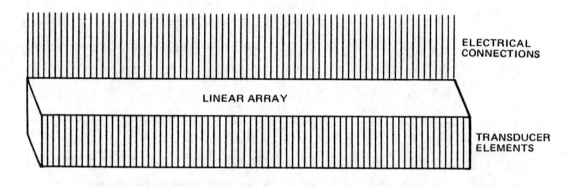

Figure 3-7. Linear Array

• Frequency Selection

The frequency of a transducer is a determining factor in its use.
Basic characteristics are affected by the need for sensitivity.
Sensitivity is related to wavelength: the higher the frequency, the
shorter the wavelength; the shorter the wavelength, the higher the

sensitivity. Transducer frequency and crystal thickness are also related. The higher the frequency, the thinner the crystal. For example, a 15-MHz transducer has a crystal only about 0.007 inch (0.2 mm), which is fragile for contact testing. If such a crystal were used in the contact testing technique, the near zone length would have to be evaluated. It is possible to place a "delay line" or "standoff" on the end of a contact probe to compensate for the near zone. In this way, the sound beam entering the test object would be limited to the far zone and would therefore be useful. Immersion testing makes this compensation with the water path. For this reason, the immersion testing technique would be the better choice when testing conditions require the use of a 15-MHz or higher-frequency transducer. However, contact transducers of 25 MHz and higher are commercially available. Other considerations are:

—   The higher the frequency of a transducer, the narrower (less beam spread) the sound beam and the greater the sensitivity and resolution, but the attenuation is also greatest and the penetration is poor.

—   The lower the frequency of a transducer, the deeper the penetration and the less the attenuation; but the greater the beam spread, the less the sensitivity and resolution.

—   At any given frequency, the larger the transducer, the narrower the sound beam and the greater the sensitivity.

Couplants

●   General

One of the practical problems in ultrasonic testing is the

transmission of the ultrasonic energy from the source into the test specimen. If a transducer is placed in contact with the surface of a dry part, very little energy is transmitted through the interface into the material because of the presence of air between the transducer and the test material. The air causes a great difference in acoustic impedance (impedance mismatch) at the interface.

A couplant is used between the transducer face and the test surface to ensure efficient sound transmission from transducer to test article. The couplant, as the name implies, couples the transducer ultrasonically to the test specimen by filling the minor irregularities of the test surface and by excluding all air from between the transducer and the test surface. The couplant can be any of a vast variety of liquids, semiliquids, pastes, and even some solids, that will satisfy the following requirements.

—   A couplant wets (fully contacts) both the surface of the test specimen and the face of the transducer and excludes all air from between them.

—   A couplant is easy to apply.

—   A couplant is homogeneous and free of air bubbles, or solid particles in the case of a nonsolid.

—   A couplant is harmless to the test specimen and transducer.

—   A couplant has a tendency to stay on the test surface, but is easy to remove.

- A couplant has an acoustic impedance value between the impedance value of the transducer face and the impedance value of the test specimen, preferably approaching that of the test surface.

● Immersion Couplant Selection

In immersion testing, nothing more than clean, deaerated tap water with a corrosion inhibitor and a wetting agent is used for a couplant. For operator comfort, the water temperature is usually maintained at 70°F (21°C) by automatic controls. Wetting agents are added to the water to ensure that the surface is thoroughly wet, thereby eliminating air bubbles.

● Contact Couplant Selection

In contact testing, the choice of couplant depends primarily on the test conditions; i.e., the condition of the test surface (rough or smooth), the temperature of the test surface, and the position of the test surface (horizontal, slanted, or vertical).

One part gelatin (cellulose) with two parts water and a wetting agent is often used on relatively smooth, horizontal surfaces. For slightly rough surfaces, light oils (such as engine oil) may also be used. Rough surfaces, hot surfaces, and vertical surfaces require the use of a heavier or special-purpose couplants. In all cases, the couplant selected must be as thin as possible and allow for consistent, effective results. Couplant manufacturers offer a wide variety of special couplants.

Standard Reference Blocks

- General

In ultrasonic testing, all discontinuity indications are compared to indications received from testing a reference standard. The reference standard may be any one of many reference blocks or sets of blocks specified for a given test. Ultrasonic standard reference blocks, often called test blocks, are used in ultrasonic testing to calibrate the ultrasonic equipment and to evaluate the discontinuity indications received from the part under test. Calibrating does two things: it verifies that the instrument/transducer combination is performing as required, and it establishes a sensitivity or gain setting at which all discontinuities of the size specified, or larger, should be detected. Evaluation of discontinuities within the test specimen is accomplished by comparing their indications with the indication received from artificial discontinuities of known size and at the same sound path In a standard reference block of the same material. Remember, other factors (type of reflector, orientation of the reflector, etc.) affect this relative "size" estimate.

Standard test blocks are made from stock which has been carefully selected and ultrasonically inspected and which meets predetermined standards of sound attenuation, grain size, and heat-treat. Discontinuities can be represented by flat-bottomed holes (FBHs) which are carefully drilled, side-drilled holes (SDH's) or notches. Test blocks are made and tested with painstaking care so that the only discontinuity present is the one that was added intentionally. Three such sets of standard reference blocks are: (1) the area amplitude blocks; (2) the distance amplitude blocks and; (3) the ASTM basic set of blocks that combine area amplitude and distance amplitude blocks in one set. To streamline the text, refer to Table 3-2 to convert to metric units as we continue our discussion of reference blocks.

Table 3-2. Metric Equivalents

Fraction (inch)	Metric Equivalent (mm)
1/64	0.4
2/64; 1/32	0.8
3/64	1.2
4/64; 1/16	1.6
5/64	2.0
6/64; 3/32	2.4
7/64	2.8
8/64; 1/8	3.2

● Area Amplitude Block Set

This set consists of 8 blocks, each 3-3/4 inches (95.3 mm) long and 1-15/16 inches (49.2 mm) square. A 3/4 inch deep (19 mm), flat-bottomed hole is drilled in the bottom center of each block. The hole diameters are 1/64 inch in the No. 1 block through 8/64 inch in the No. 8 block, as illustrated in Figure 3-8. As implied, the block numbers refer to the FBH diameter; e.g., a No. 3 block has a 3/64 inch diameter flat-bottomed hole. Similar area amplitude reference blocks are made from 2-inch-diameter (50.8 mm) round stock.

Area amplitude blocks provide a means of checking the linearity of the test system. They confirm that the amplitude (height) of the indication in the display increases in proportion to the increase in size of the discontinuity.

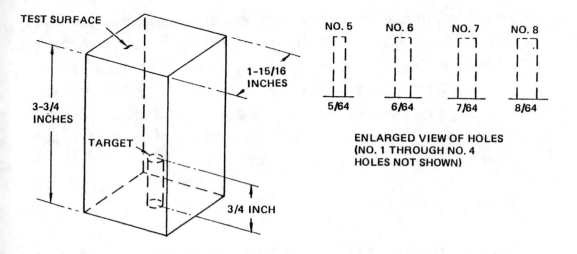

Figure 3-8. Area Amplitude Reference Blocks

- Distance Amplitude Block Set

This set of blocks consists of nineteen 2-inch-diameter (50.8 mm) cylindrical blocks, all with 3/4 inch deep (19 mm) flat-bottomed holes of the same diameter drilled in the center at one end. These blocks are of different lengths to provide sound-path distances of 1/16 inch to 5-3/4 inches (146.1 mm) from the test surface to the flat-bottomed hole. Sets with 3/64, 5/64, or 8/64 inch-diameter holes are available. The sound-path distances in each set are: 1/16 inch, 1/8 inch through 1 inch in 1/8-inch increments, and 1-1/4 inches (131.8 mm) through 5-3/4 inches (146.1 mm) in 1/2-inch (12.7 mm) increments.

Distance amplitude blocks serve as a reference by which the size of discontinuities at varying sound-path distances within the test material may be evaluated. They also serve as a reference for establishing the sensitivity or gain of the test system so that the system will display readable indications for all discontinuities of a given size, but will not flood the screen with indications that are of no interest. On instruments so equipped, these blocks are used to set the STC (sensitivity time control) or DAC (distance amplitude correction) so that a discontinuity of a given size will produce an indication of the same amplitude regardless of its sound-path distance from the examination surface.

- Basic Block Set

The ASTM basic set consists of 10 blocks which are 2 inches in diameter (50.8 mm) that have 3/4 inch deep (19 mm) flat-bottomed holes drilled in the center at one end. One block has a 3/64 inch-diameter FBH and a sound-path distance of 3 inches (76.2 mm) from the test surface to the flat-bottomed hole. The next 7 blocks each have a 5/64-inch FBH but sound-path distances are 1/8, 1/4, 1/2, 3/4, 1-1/2, 3, and 6 inches (3.2, 6.3, 12.7, 19, 38.1, 76.2, and 152.4 mm) from the test surface to the FBH. The 2 remaining blocks each have an 8/64 inch diameter FBH and sound-path distances of 3 inches (76.2 mm) and 6 inches (152.4 mm). In this basic set the 3 (No. 3, 5, and 8) blocks with the 3-inch (76.2 mm) sound-path distance provide the area amplitude relationship, and the 7 blocks with the 5/64 inch diameter FBH (No. 5) and varying sound-path distances provide the distance amplitude relationship.

It is important that the test block material be the same or similar to that of the test specimen. Alloy content, heat-treatment, degree of hot or cold working from forging, rolling, etc., all affect the acoustical properties of the material. If test blocks of identical material are not available, they must be similar in ultrasound attenuation, surface condition, velocity, and acoustic impedance.

- Other Blocks

  The IIW (International Institute of Welding) reference block and the miniature angle beam field calibration block (Rompas block) shown in Figure 3-9 are examples of other reference standards in common use.

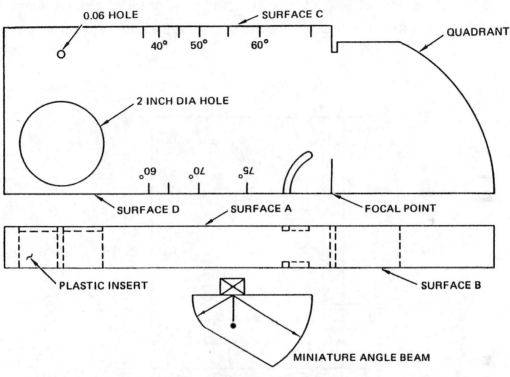

Figure 3-9. Other Reference Blocks

  For irregularly-shaped articles, it is often necessary to make one of the test articles into a reference standard by adding artificial discontinuities in the form of flat-bottomed holes, saw cuts, notches, cracks, etc. In some cases, these artificial discontinuities can be placed so that they will be removed by subsequent machining of the article. In other cases, a special individual calibration technique is developed by carefully studying an article ultrasonically and then verifying the detection of discontinuities in the article by destructive investigation. The results of the study then become the basis for the testing standard.

Another block that is used for calibration is the ASME piping calibration block as illustrated in Figure 3-10. This block is specified in the ASME Boiler and Pressure Vessel Code and is used by various industries. Many specialty calibration blocks exist for various material types, discontinuity orientations and applications.

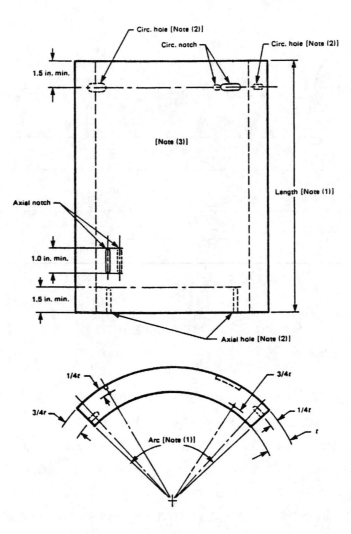

Figure 3-10. ASME Piping Calibration Block

- Mockups

In some cases real flaws are implanted at critical locations in a mockup to simulate the ultrasonic examination that will later be conducted on actual components. Unlike reference and calibration blocks, these mockups are often used as a capability demonstration to qualify UT procedures and personnel. As shown in Figure 3-11 and 3-12, mockups and other intentionally flawed specimens are available from several commercial sources including the publisher of this text.

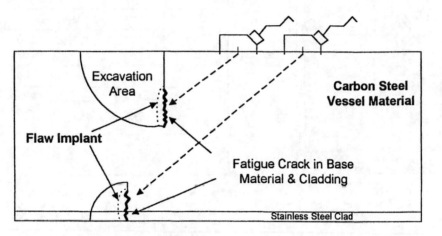

Figure 3-11. Typical Mockup of Fatigue Crack Implant in Thick Vessel Material

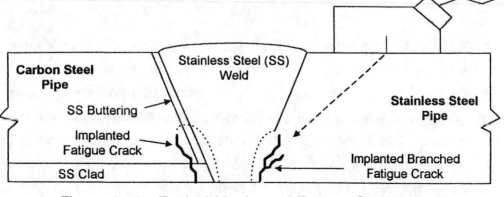

Figure 3-12. Typical Mockup of Fatigue Cracks in Dissimilar Metal Piping Weld

Display

Figure 3-13 shows a typical ultrasonic contact test setup and the resulting CRT display. Notice the position of the displayed indications on the screen in relation to the actual positions of the test piece front surface, discontinuity, and back surface.

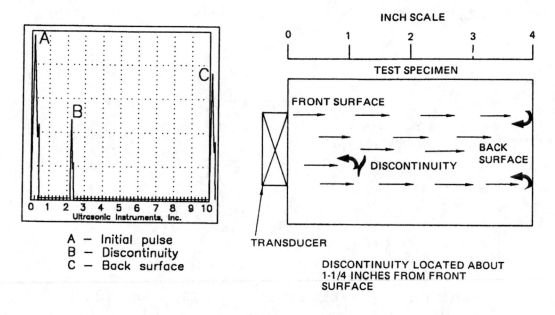

Figure 3-13. Typical Contact Ultrasonic Test Display

The CRT is divided into *horizontal screen divisions* located below the horizontal sweep. There are normally 10 *major* screen divisions, each broken down into 5 *minor* divisions. The horizontal screen divisions are used as relative units of time or distance. We can adjust the ultrasonic instrument so that these screen divisions represent a specific distance (or time) between the front surface reflection and the back surface reflection, in inches, cm., etc. There may be 5 or 10 horizontal screen divisions, depending on the instrument manufacturer. These are used to compare indication amplitude.

In Figure 3-13, the indications were adjusted to position the initial pulse, or front surface indication, on the 0 major screen division. The back surface indication is on the 10th major screen division. The discontinuity indication appears just to the right of the 2nd major screen division (at 2.2 screen divisions). The indication positions were accomplished by varying two controls on the instrument; the DELAY and the SWEEP LENGTH, MATERIAL CALIBRATION, or RANGE controls.

Basic Instrument Operation

● General

A cathode-ray tube (CRT) is often used to display ultrasonic indications in a manner similar to a television picture tube. Figure 3-14 shows a typical cathode-ray tube and its electron gun. This tube comes in many sizes and shapes. It is made of specially-tested glass that is constructed with a screen at one end for the picture display. The screen is coated with material called a phosphor compound which varies in composition to produce various brightnesses, colors, and time persistence. The phosphor compound glows and produces light when bombarded by high-speed electrons directed at the screen from the electron gun in the base of the tube.

At the opposite end of the tube, electrons are produced in the electron gun. The electrons are emitted from a hot filament similar to the filament in an ordinary light bulb. By electromagnetic means, these electrons are accelerated and focused to form a beam the size of a pinhead when it strikes the phosphor screen. The position of the spot on the screen is altered by changing the direction of the electron beam. Changing the direction of the electron beam is accomplished by changing the electrical charge on the horizontal and vertical deflection plates.

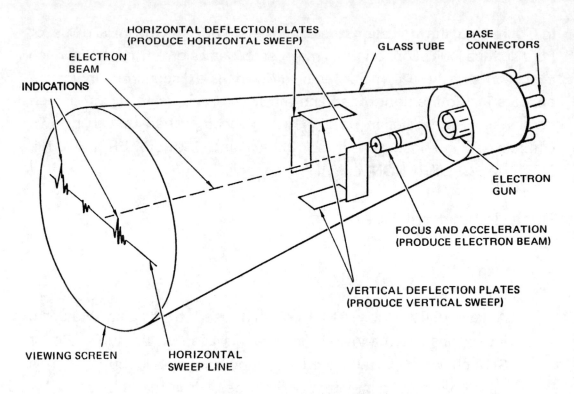

HORIZONTAL DEFLECTION PLATES
(PRODUCE HORIZONTAL SWEEP)

BASE
CONNECTORS

GLASS TUBE

ELECTRON
BEAM

INDICATIONS

ELECTRON
GUN

FOCUS AND ACCELERATION
(PRODUCE ELECTRON BEAM)

VERTICAL DEFLECTION PLATES
(PRODUCE VERTICAL SWEEP)

VIEWING SCREEN

HORIZONTAL
SWEEP LINE

Figure 3-14. Typical Cathode-Ray Tube (CRT)

In ultrasonic testing, the CRT usually shows a bright horizontal line when there is no signal received. This horizontal line is called the sweep or baseline. An electronic circuit energizes the horizontal deflection plates to cause the electron beam to sweep from the left edge of the screen to the right edge at a certain fixed speed. As soon as the beam reaches the right edge, it is caused to return to the left edge at a very high speed, too fast to be seen on the screen. In operation, the electron beam draws a line of light across the screen. The line length is a measure of the time required for the spot on the screen to move from left to right.

Distance may be determined when time and speed are known. The distance along the line represents the lapse of time since the initial pulse (sound entry surface) and this lapse of time multiplied by speed equals distance from the sound entry surface. By adjusting the sweep speed of the electron beam, the baseline may be adjusted to represent a particular distance.

When a signal is relayed to the CRT from the transducer, a voltage is applied to the vertical deflection plates, causing a vertical indication to appear from the line. When the transducer receives signals reflected from the test piece front and back surface, voltages are again applied to the vertical deflection plates and the front surface indication appears first and the back surface indication appears some time later on the baseline. The spacing between these indications is a measure of the sound-path distance between the surfaces.

Digitized displays are also utilized and offer great advantages in size and weight over the typical CRT described above. Additionally, digitization of the data permits data transfer to computer-based systems for further interpretation, evaluation, multiscan display, and data archiving.

●   Sweep Delay

The DELAY control of the instrument permits the baseline and the indications on it to be shifted either to the right or to the left while the spacing between the indications remains constant. Figure 3-15 shows the result of adjusting the DELAY control to shift the baseline to the left in order to see the indications related to the material under test (see Figure 3-13 for test setup).

In Figure 3-15, the operator first picked up the front surface indication (which is also the initial pulse in this example) and the discontinuity indication. By adjusting the DELAY, the front surface indication is moved to the far left bringing the discontinuity and back surface indications into view. Notice that the distance between the first two indications has not changed.

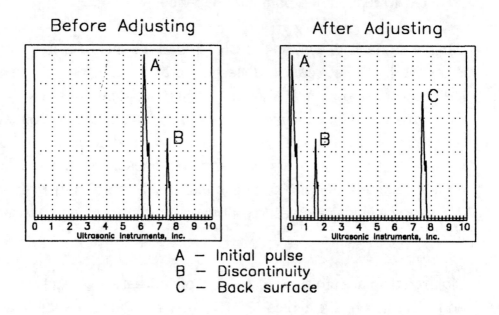

A — Initial pulse
B — Discontinuity
C — Back surface

Figure 3-15. Sweep Delay Adjustment

● Sweep Length (Range)

Now that the delay has been adjusted the RANGE adjustment must be considered. The operator may wish to display the front and back surface indications so that the distance relationship and horizontal positions on the screen is directly related to the actual dimension of the test piece. To do this, the horizontal trace or baseline is expanded or contracted to change the distance between the indications displayed. The discontinuity indication is always located in the same relative position with respect to the front and back surface indications.

- The expansion or contraction of the baseline is away from or toward the left side of the screen. That is, if the DELAY is set so that the start of the desired presentation is at the left side of the screen, adjustment of the RANGE moves the right-hand indications away from or toward the left-hand indication. The DELAY control also makes it possible to view the responses from any desired segment of the sweep. In effect, the DELAY control allows the viewing screen to be moved along the sound path of the part. In conjunction with the RANGE control, the DELAY makes it possible to examine a magnified segment of the part by spreading the segment across the entire width of the display.

- Figure 3-16 shows the CRT presentation before and after the RANGE has been adjusted to expand the view of the entire part across the screen with the front surface and back surface indications aligned with the 0 and 10th screen divisions respectively. Assume that the CRT represents 10 inches (254 mm) full screen width (FSW). The discontinuity is located at 2.2 screen division which represents 2.2 inches (55.9 mm) from the sound entry surface.

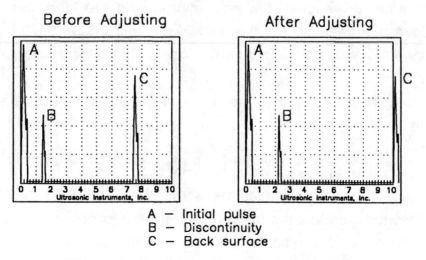

Before Adjusting   After Adjusting

A — Initial pulse
B — Discontinuity
C — Back surface

Figure 3-16. Sweep Length Adjustment

— Two controls, the DELAY and the RANGE, regulate how much of the test part is presented at one time on the screen and what portion, if not the whole, of the part is presented.

● Summary

After the instrument is turned on, allowed to warm up, and/or has completed the self-test, the first adjustments made on the instrument concern scale illumination, baseline intensity focus, horizontal positioning, and vertical positioning. The power ON switch may contain a control for the brightness of the scale scribed on the CRT screen overlay. This brightness is considered a matter of personal choice. The intensity control determines the brightness of the spot moving across the screen to form the sweep line. Sweep line intensity is kept at a minimum with no bright spot at either end. The astigmatism and focus controls adjust the sharpness of the screen presentation. The horizontal positioning control determines the starting point of the sweep line on the CRT, which is usually at the left edge of the screen. The vertical positioning control raises and lowers the sweep line or baseline to coincide with the screen graticules. The exact procedures to operate and adjust the many controls of various ultrasonic instruments are described in the operation manual for the individual instrument. The precise capabilities of each instrument is contained in the same source.

A simplified block diagram of a typical A-scan pulse-echo ultrasonic testing instrument is shown in Figure 3-17. The timer or rate generator is the heart of the system. In the contact testing setup illustrated, the energizing pulse from the pulse unit is routed to the receiver amplifier unit at the same time that it is sent to the transducer so that the initial pulse and the front surface indication occur at nearly the same time. In an immersion testing setup, the

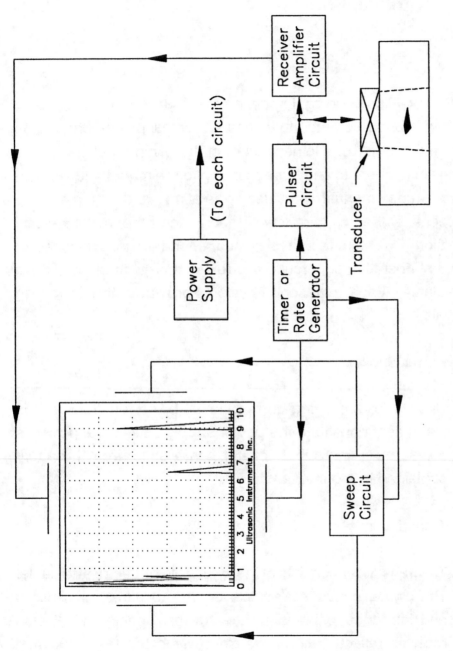

Figure 3-17. Pulse-Echo Unit, Block Diagram

initial pulse and the front surface indication are separated by the water travel distance to the test piece.

Pulse-Echo Instruments

• General

All makes of pulse-echo equipment have similar electronics circuitry and provide basic common functions. A typical pulse-echo unit is shown in Figure 3-18. Nomenclature of the given functions varies from one instrument to another according to the manufacturer. The manufacturer's manual provides operation and maintenance instructions for the unit, a review of theory, and other more specific information. Manufacturers' recommendations concerning instrument operation supersede this text in the event of conflicting information. Each ultrasonic system provides the following essentials:

– Power Supply

Circuits for supplying current for all basic functions of the instrument constitute the power supply. Electrical power is served from line supply or, for some units, from a battery contained in the instrument.

– Transducer

The transducer consists of the crystal, its housing, and cable. The crystal converts electrical energy to ultrasonic energy and introduces vibrations into the test specimen. It also receives reflected vibrations from within the test specimen and converts them into electrical signals for amplification and display.

– Pulser/Receiver

The pulser, or pulse generator, is the source of short high-energy bursts of electrical energy (triggered by the timer) which are applied to the transducer. Return pulses from the test specimen are received, amplified, and routed to the display unit.

– Display/Timer

The display is usually a CRT or a digitized display with a sweep generator and the controls required to provide a visual image of the signals received from the test specimen. The timer is the source of all timing signals to the pulser and is sometimes referred to as the rate generator or clock.

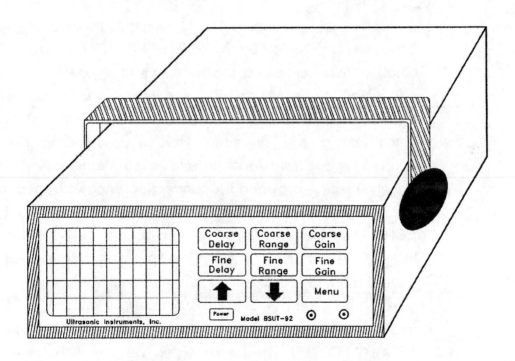

Figure 3-18. Typical Pulse-Echo Unit

•   Controls

Controls are provided for the various systems of the instrument, such as power supply, pulser, receiver, timer, and display. The nomenclature used in the following description of the controls may vary from one type of unit to another.

–   Power Supply

The power supply is usually controlled by an ON-OFF switch and a fuse. After turning power on, there are certain time-delay devices which protect circuit elements during instrument warm-up.

–   Pulser/Receiver

The pulse of ultrasonic energy transmitted into the test specimen is adjusted by the PULSE LENGTH control. For single-transducer testing, the transmit and receive circuits are connected to one jack on the same transducer. For double-transducer testing, called through-transmission or pitch-and-catch testing, a T (transmit) jack is provided to permit connecting one transducer for use as a transmitter and an R (receive) jack is provided for connecting another transducer for receiving only. A MODE switch for THRU or PULSE-ECHO transmission is provided for control of the T and R jacks. A selector for a range of operating frequencies is usually marked FREQUENCY with the available frequencies given in megahertz. Gain controls usually consist of FINE and COARSE sensitivity selectors or one control marked SENSITIVITY. For a cleaner video display with low-level noise minimized, a REJECT control is provided.

– Display/Timer

The display controls and their functions for the display unit are as follows:

- Vertical - Controls the vertical position of the indications displayed.

- Horizontal - Controls the horizontal position of the indications displayed.

- Intensity - Varies the brightness of the display as desired.

- Focus - Adjusts the focus of the trace.

- Astigmatism - Corrects for distortion or astigmatism introduced by changing transmit time of the electron beam across the oscilloscope screen.

- Power - Turns power on and off for entire unit.

- Scale Illumination - Adjusts illumination of the grid lines when provided.

Timer circuits usually consist of a pulse repetition rate device which controls the rate at which pulses are generated to other circuits. Pulse repetition rate is varied to suit the material and thickness of the test specimen. The DELAY control is also used to position the initial pulse on the left side of the display screen with a back surface reflection, or multiples of back surface reflections, visible on the right side of the screen.

— Other Controls

Other controls, which are refinements not always provided, include the following:

- DAC or STC

  DAC (Distance Amplitude Correction), STC (Sensitivity Time Control), and other like units called TCG (Time Corrected Gain), or TVG (Time Varied Gain) are used to compensate for a drop in amplitude of signals from reflectors of long sound paths within the test specimen.

- Damping

  The pulse duration is shortened by the DAMPING control which adjusts the length of the wave train applied to the transducer. Resolution is improved by increasing the damping.

- Display Selector

  The DISPLAY SELECTOR switch is used to select the desired type of display, RADIO FREQUENCY or VIDEO.

- Gated Alarm

  Gated alarm units enable the use of automatic alarms when discontinuities are detected. This is accomplished by setting up specific gated or zoned areas within the test specimen. Signals appearing within these gates may be monitored automatically to operate visual or audible alarms. These signals are also passed on to process feedback control devices. Gated alarm units usually have three controls as follows:

-- Start or Delay

The gate START or DELAY control is used for adjustment of the location of the leading edge of the gate.

-- Length or Width

The gate LENGTH or WIDTH control is used for adjustment of the width of the gate or the location of the gate trailing edge.

-- Alarm Level or Threshold

The alarm LEVEL or THRESHOLD control is used for adjustment of the gate's vertical threshold (either + or -) to turn on signal lights or to activate an alarm.

• A-scan Equipment

The A-scan system is a data presentation technique that displays the returned signal amplitude from the material under test as illustrated in Figure 3-19. The horizontal baseline indicates elapsed time (from left to right), and the vertical deflection shows signal amplitudes. For a given ultrasonic velocity in the specimen, the sweep can be calibrated directly across the screen in terms of sound-path distance or depth of penetration into the sample. Conversely, when the dimensions of the sample are known, the sweep time may be used to determine ultrasonic velocities. The height of the indications represent the intensities of the reflected sound beams. These may be used to determine the relative size of the discontinuity, the depth or distance to the discontinuity from the front or back surface, the sound beam spread, and other factors. The chief advantage of this equipment is that it provides amplitude information needed to evaluate the relative size and position of the discontinuity.

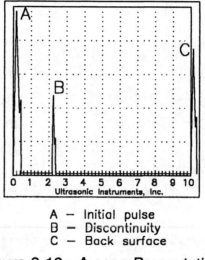

A — Initial pulse
B — Discontinuity
C — Back surface

Figure 3-19. A-scan Presentation

• B-scan Equipment

The B-scan system shown in Figure 3-20 is particularly useful where the distribution, shape and location of large discontinuities within a sample cross section is of interest. A chief advantage of the B-scan equipment is that a cross-sectional view of the sample and the discontinuities within it are displayed. In computerized high-speed scanning, the cross-section image is used to evaluate several cross sections of the sample in the area(s) containing the discontinuity(s).

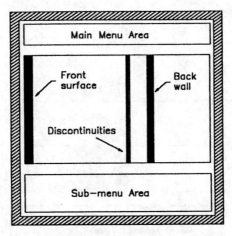

Typical Computer Monitor B—scan Display
Illustrates the depth (sound path) and
length of the discontinuities.

Figure 3-20. B-scan Presentation

• C-scan Equipment

C-scan equipment displays the test article and associated discontinuities in a plan (or top) view. The C-scan recording indicates the projected length and width of the discontinuity and the outline of the test specimen as if viewed from directly above the specimen. The C-scan recording indicates the depth of the discontinuity in the test specimen. The same signals that generate the indications on the A-scan produce a change on the C-scan recording. The front and back surface signals from the specimen are eliminated from the recording by the instrument gating circuits, and the alarm sensitivity control setting determines the amplitude of the signal (indication) required to produce a change on the recording. Commonly used displays are high-resolution color computer monitors and liquid crystal displays (LCD's). The data can be readily printed on a multicolor printer or stored on magnetic or optical media. Figure 3-21 shows a C-scan presentation.

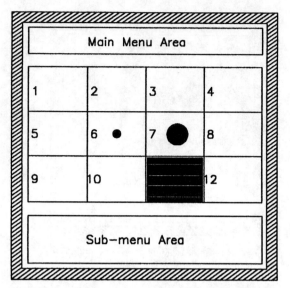

Typical Computer Monitor C—scan Display
Illustrates the use of 12 gates simultaneously.

Figure 3-21. C-scan Presentation

● Digital Thickness Gauges

The digital thickness gauge is a specialized A-scan instrument that utilizes the DAC to determine when the first indication of interest returns to the search unit. Time is kept by an electronic counter which displays the sound-path distance digitally on the LCD. The operation is straightforward and is based on the velocity of the material under test (range control) and the thickness of a standard (delay setting). Surface condition problems can cause these types of instruments to yield misinformation. Often times a digitized typical A-scan presentation is presented with the LCD digital display to better inform the operator of test conditions. Two typical digital thickness gauges are illustrated in Figure 3-22.

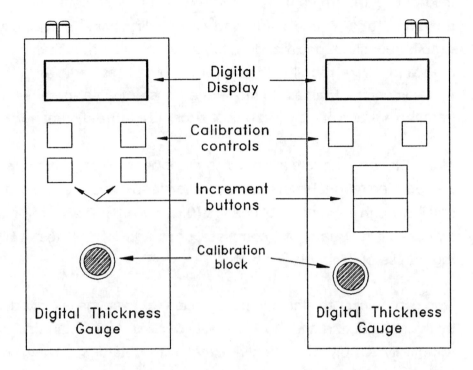

Figure 3-22. Digital Thickness Gauges

Computer-Based Ultrasonics

- General

There are many types of components that can be utilized to design
and assemble a system. As shown in Figure 3-23, many ultrasonic
systems are composed of a personal computer, a high-resolution
color monitor, modular ultrasonic circuit components, a scanner and
scanner controller, an immersion tank outfitted with a carriage and
bridge, and a search unit manipulator, and often, an in-tank
turntable.

Generally probes mounted in scanners similar to the one on the following page are capable of three axes of movement. They can move in the X, Y, and Z (up and down) directions individually or simultaneously. Specialized systems can provide movement in five axes and utilize robotics to load and unload test articles. These systems can be "trained" to move at a constant water-path distance from the surface of a curved object such as a large-diameter vessel.

Most of these scanners are driven by stepper motors, but some can be operated manually if necessary. The stepper motors can provide small enough increments of change (0.01" which is 0.25 mm or less) to essentially guarantee complete coverage of the test object, regardless of the probe chosen.

One can quickly see that the possibilities for systems is limited only by the imagination and the availability of resources. Manufacturers will gladly supply the potential client with catalogs. They would surely entertain customizing a system for your application should you prefer.

Many systems can display the A-scan, B-scan, and C-scan information simultaneously. Such a feature is a useful aid to the data analysts.

The ultrasonic systems described so far have been associated with immersion systems. It must be said that many of the same data presentations and displays are an integral part of systems utilizing portable scanners such as those used for the testing of pipe, vessels, storage tanks, and similar components. Much NDT done in the field is on as-found components, so it is important that we adapt our test apparatus to the actual component configurations.

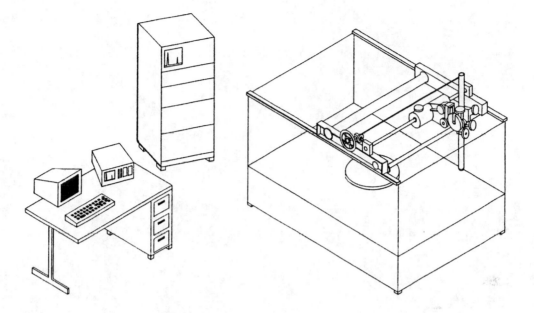

Figure 3-23.   Computer-Based System

Ultrasonic systems and scanners, their design, attachments and drive mechanisms range from simple to complex. Consequently, so do their costs. It is beyond the scope of this text to describe the various types of equipment available. There are organizations that will design a specialized system to your specifications or perform application analysis.

CHAPTER 4: TECHNIQUE AND APPLICATIONS

TABLE OF CONTENTS

TABLE OF CONTENTS (CONT'D.)

LIST OF FIGURES

LIST OF FIGURES (CONT'D.)

CHAPTER 4

TECHNIQUE AND APPLICATIONS

General

Ultrasonic testing, like other NDT testing techniques, follows a set pattern of events that are designed to give consistent results. Ultrasonic testing consists of the following basic steps.

- Calibration of the test system
- Performance of the test
- Interpretation of results

The paragraphs that follow outline these basic steps.

Testing Procedures

- General

  The type of test and technique required for a particular component is usually specified in a test procedure that tells the operator the type discontinuities one is to look for, the type of test required to locate the discontinuities, the definition of limits of acceptability and gives other basic facts pertinent to the test. Either the contact or immersion technique can be utilized in the test procedure. It is the responsibility of the operator to follow the procedure. The paragraphs that follow are intended to familiarize the operator with basic steps that are required to conduct satisfactory ultrasonic tests.

Prior to any ultrasonic test it is important to verify that the test instrument is internally (or electronically) calibrated. This ensures the proper performance of the test instrument and the linearity of the response of the instrument to discontinuities of different sizes and sound-path distances.

- Calibration of the Test System

Calibration of the testing system is a vital step in the test procedure. Calibrating is the adjustment of the equipment controls so that the operator can be sure that the instrument will detect the discontinuities one is expected to find. Calibrating the system consists of setting up the instrument system as it is to be used in the test and adjusting the controls to give an adequate response to discontinuities of known size and sound-path distance in specific reference standards. The type, size, and position of the artificial discontinuities are specified in the test specification.

- Performance of the Test

Once the ultrasonic system is calibrated, the actual testing can begin. Limited access to the instrument controls are permitted during actual testing since adjusting certain controls negate the calibration and may require recalibration.

Ultrasonic tests are accomplished with one of two basic techniques: contact or immersion testing. In contact testing, the transducer is placed in direct contact with the test specimen with a thin liquid film used as a couplant. On some contact units, plastic wedges, wear plates, or flexible membranes are mounted over the face of the search unit. The display from a contact search unit usually shows the initial pulse and the front surface reflection very close together. In immersion testing, a waterproof transducer is used at some distance from the test specimen and the ultrasonic beam is transmitted into the material through a water path or column. Because of the reduced velocity of ultrasound in water, the water distance appears on the display with a fairly wide space between the initial pulse and the front surface reflection. The particular procedure to be used is specified in the test procedure.

- Interpretation of Results

Once the ultrasonic test has been performed, the results must be interpreted. Many factors must be taken into consideration in interpreting the results of an ultrasonic test. These are outlined later in this chapter.

Immersion Testing

- General

Any one of several techniques may be used in immersion testing: (a) the immersion technique where both the transducer and the test specimen are immersed in water; (b) the bubbler or squirter technique where the sound beam is transmitted through a column of flowing water; and (c) the wheel transducer technique where the transducer is mounted in the axle of a liquid-filled tire that rolls on the test surface. An adaptation of the wheel transducer technique is a unit with the transducer mounted in the top of a water-filled tube. A flexible membrane on the lower end of the tube couples the unit to the test surface. In all of these techniques, a further refinement is the use of focused transducers that concentrate the sound beam (much like light beams are concentrated when passed through a magnifying glass). The bubbler and wheel transducer techniques are illustrated in Figure 4-1.

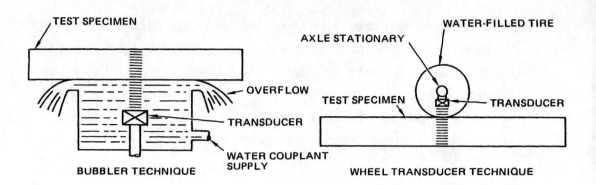

Figure 4-1. Bubbler and Wheel Transducer Techniques

- Immersion Techniques

In the immersion technique, both the transducer and the test specimen are immersed in water. The sound beam is directed through the water into the material using either a straight beam technique for generating longitudinal waves or one of the many angle beam techniques for generating shear waves in the test article. In many automatic scanning operations, focused beams are used to detect near surface discontinuities or to define minute discontinuities with the concentrated sound beam.

The transducers usually used in immersion testing are straight beam units that accomplish both straight and angle beam testing through manipulation and control of the sound beam direction. The water-path distance must be considered in immersion testing. This is the distance between the face of the transducer and the surface of the test specimen. This distance is usually adjusted so that the time required to send the sound beam through the water is greater than the time required for the sound to travel through the test specimen. When done properly, the second front surface reflection will not appear in the display between the first front and first back surface reflections. In water, sound velocity is about 1/4 that of aluminum or steel; therefore, 1 inch (25.4 mm) of water path will appear on the monitor as equal to 4 inches (101.6 mm) of sound path in steel. As a rule of thumb, position the transducer so that the water distance is equal to 1/4 the thickness of the part plus 1/4 inch (6.4 mm). The correct water-path distance is particularly important when the test area shown in the display is gated for automatic signaling and recording operations. The water-path distance is carefully set to clear the test area of unwanted signals that cause confusion and possible misinterpretation. Figure 4-2 illustrates the relationship between the actual water path and the display.

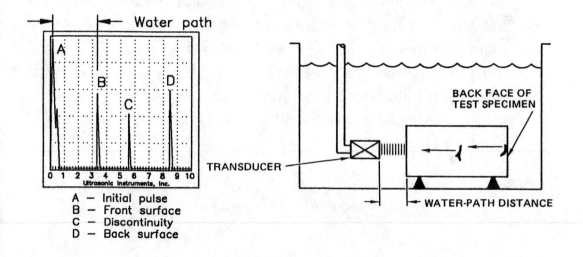

Figure 4-2. Water-Path Distance Adjustment

● Bubbler Techniques

The bubbler technique is a variation of the immersion method. In the bubbler technique the sound beam is projected through a water column into the test specimen. The bubbler is usually used with an

4-5

automated system for high-speed scanning of plate, sheet, strip, cylindrical forms, and other regularly-shaped parts. The ultrasound is projected into the material through a column of flowing water, and is directed in a normal direction (perpendicular) to the test surface to produce longitudinal waves or is adjusted at an angle to the surface to produce shear waves.

- Wheel Transducer Techniques

The wheel transducer technique is an aspect of the immersion method in that the ultrasound is projected through a water-filled tire into the test specimen. The transducer, mounted in the wheel axle, is held in a fixed position, while the wheel and tire rotate freely. The wheel may be mounted on a mobile apparatus that runs across the material, or it may be mounted on a stationary fixture where the material is moved past it. Figure 4-3 illustrates the stationary and the moving-wheel transducer. The position and angle of the transducer mounting on the wheel axle may be constructed to project straight beams as shown in Figure 4-3, or to project angled beams as shown in Figure 4-4.

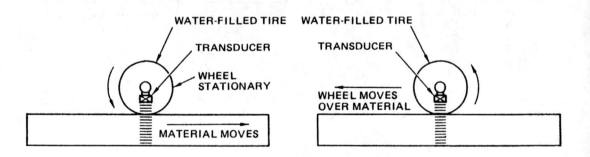

Figure 4-3. Stationary and Moving-Wheel Transducer

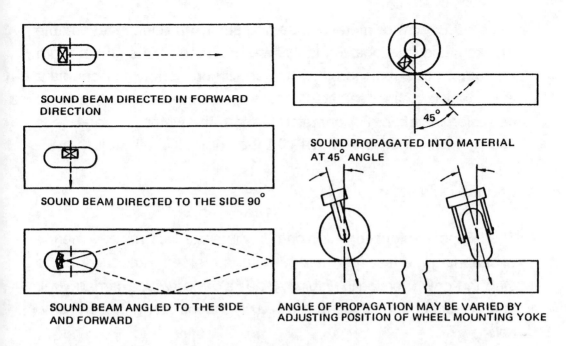

SOUND BEAM DIRECTED IN FORWARD
DIRECTION

SOUND BEAM DIRECTED TO THE SIDE 90°

SOUND BEAM ANGLED TO THE SIDE
AND FORWARD

SOUND PROPAGATED INTO MATERIAL
AT 45° ANGLE

45°

ANGLE OF PROPAGATION MAY BE VARIED BY
ADJUSTING POSITION OF WHEEL MOUNTING YOKE

Figure 4-4. Wheel Transducer Angular Capabilities

Ultrasonic Tank and Bridge/Manipulator

● General

Ultrasonic tanks and bridge/manipulators are necessary equipment
for high-speed scanning of immersed test specimens. Modern units
consist of a bridge and manipulator mounted over a fairly large
water tank. Drive power units move the bridge along the tank side
rails while traversing power units move the manipulator from side to
side along the bridge. Most of these units are automated, although
they can be manually operated.

● Ultrasonic Tank

The ultrasonic tank may be of any size or shape required to
accommodate the test specimen. Coverage of the specimen by

1 foot (30.5 cm) or more of water is usually sufficient. Adjustable brackets and rotational turntables are provided on the tank bottom for support and rotation of the test specimen. The water couplant in the tank is clean, deaerated water containing a wetting agent and corrosion inhibitor. For operator comfort, the water temperature is usually maintained at 70°F (21°C) by automatic controls.

- Bridge/Manipulator

The bridge/manipulator unit is primarily intended to provide a means of scanning the test specimen with an immersed transducer. The stripped-down version in Figure 4-5 has a bridge with a carriage unit at each end so the bridge may be easily moved along the tank side rails.

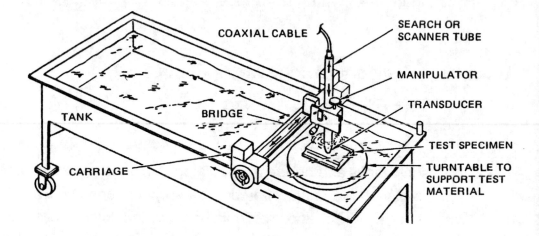

Figure 4-5. Bridge/Manipulator

The manipulator is mounted on a traversing mechanism which allows movement of the manipulator from side to side. The traversing mechanism is an integral component of the bridge assembly. The search tube is usually held rigid, as illustrated, at right angles to the surface of the test specimen. Locking knobs are provided on the manipulator to allow positioning of the search tube in two planes for angle beam testing. When the equipment is automated, electric motors are added to power the bridge carriage, the traversing mechanism, and the up/down movement of the search tube. The pulse-echo unit and the recording unit may also be mounted on the bridge with all power cords secured overhead to allow movement of the bridge along the full length of the tank.

Typical Calibration Procedure

Frequent periodic factory (electronic) calibration of ultrasonic testing units is required to establish the linearity of displayed indications and to ensure proper instrument performance. Once the equipment is electronically calibrated to known standards, the operator may confidently adjust or calibrate the unit to the values of the test material. Once the test unit is electronically calibrated and calibrated to known standards, the operator can expect an accurate display of discontinuities within the test sample. When acceptance of the test sample is based on a rigid test procedure, considerable attention is given to calibration of the instrument system. Calibrating the instrument is accomplished through the use of special test blocks sometimes referred to as standard reference blocks. These blocks are made of the same material as the test sample and match the acoustical properties and dimensions of the test sample as closely as possible. Additionally, real flaws are often implanted in a mockup of the component to replicate anticipated discontinuities.

- General

  A typical calibration procedure is outlined in the paragraphs that follow. The procedures assume conditions and equipment as follows:

- Test Instrument

  Any of several commercially available pulse-echo ultrasonic testing instruments.

- Transducer

  An immersion transducer of 3/8-inch (9.5 mm) diameter with an operational frequency of 15 MHz.

- Power Source

  AC line voltage with regulation ensured by a voltage-regulating transformer.

- Immersion Tank

  Any container that holds couplant and is large enough to allow accurate positioning of the transducer and the calibration block is satisfactory.

- Couplant

  Clean, deaerated water is used as a couplant. The same water, at the same temperature, is used when comparing the responses from differing reference blocks.

- Bridge and Manipulator

  The bridge is strong enough to support the manipulator and rigid enough to allow smooth, accurate positioning of the transducer. The manipulator adequately supports the transducer and provides fine angular adjustment in two vertical planes normal to each other and in the Z-axis (up and down) direction.

- Reference Blocks

  An area amplitude set and a distance amplitude set of reference blocks are required. A basic set which combines both area and distance responses may be used; for example, the ASTM basic set consisting of 10 reference blocks.

–   Fundamental Reference Standard
When calibrating area amplitude responses of the test set, an alternate to the reference blocks described in the preceding step is the ASTM set of 15 steel balls, free of corrosion and surface marks and of ball-bearing quality, ranging in size from 1/8-inch (3.2 mm) diameter to 1-inch (25.4 mm) diameter in 1/16-inch (1.6 mm) increments. A suitable device, such as a tee pin, is necessary to hold each ball.

● Area Amplitude Check

The linear range of the instrument is determined by obtaining the ultrasonic responses from each of the area amplitude type reference blocks (the steel balls may be used as an alternate for the reference blocks) as follows:

a.   Place a No. 5 area amplitude reference block (a block containing a 5/64-inch-diameter hole) in the immersion tank with the drilled hole down. Position the transducer over the upper surface of the block, slightly off-center, at a water-path distance of 3±1/32 inches (76.2±0.8 mm) between the face of the transducer and the surface of the block. This accurate distance is obtained by using a gauge between the block and the transducer.

b.   Adjust the transducer with the manipulator to obtain a maximum indication height from the front surface reflection of the block. This indication assures that the ultrasound is perpendicular to the top surface of the block. A maximum number of back surface reflection indications serves the same purpose.

c.   Move the transducer laterally until the maximum response is received from the flat-bottomed hole.

d.   Adjust the instrument gain control until the hole indication height is 31 percent of the maximum obtainable. Do not repeat this step for the remaining blocks in the set.

e.   Replace that reference block with each of the other blocks in the set. Repeat steps "b" and "c" for each block and record the indications. Maintain a water-path distance of 3 inches (76.2 mm) for each block except for the No. 7 and No. 8 blocks which require a water distance of 6 inches (152.4 mm).

f.   Plot a curve of the recorded indications as in Figure 4-6. In the example, the points where the "curve" of responses deviates from the ideal linearity line defines the limit of linearity in the instrument. Amplitudes plotted below the "limit of linear response" (in this example) are in the linear range of the instrument and no correction is required. Amplitudes of indications above the limit of linear response are in the non-linear range and are increased to the ideal linearity curve. This is done by projecting a vertical line upward from the actual height (AH) of indication until the ideal linearity curve is intersected. The point of intersection defines the correct height (CH) of indication in percent of maximum amplitude that the instrument can display. The difference between the corrected height (CH) and the actual height (AH) is the correction factor (CF). For each indication that appears in the non-linear range a different correction factor (CF) is plotted because the deviation is not constant.

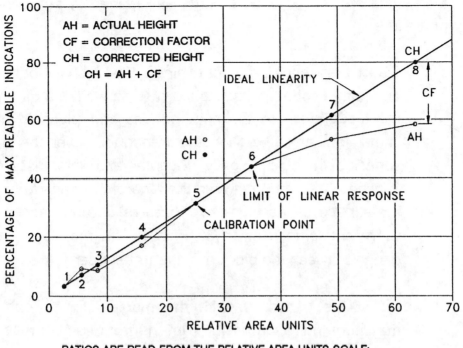

RATIOS ARE READ FROM THE RELATIVE AREA UNITS SCALE:
1/64=1; 3/64=9; 5/64=25; 8/64=64; DYNAMIC RANGE IS 64 TO 1

Figure 4-6. Typical Area Amplitude Response Curve

When the actual indication height is displayed, the corrected indication height is computed by adding the correction factor directly to the actual indication height as follows.

$$AH + CF = CH$$

• Distance Amplitude Check

The distance amplitude characteristics of the instrument are determined by obtaining the ultrasonic responses from each of the reference blocks in a set of blocks of varying sound-path distance with a 5/64 inch diameter hole in each block. The resultant indications are recorded on a curve as outlined in the following procedure:

a.   Select a reference block containing a 5/64 inch flat-bottomed hole with a sound-path distance of 3 inches (76.2 mm) from the top surface to the hole bottom and place it in the immersion tank. Position the transducer over the upper surface of the block, slightly off-center, at a water distance of 3 inches (76.2 mm) between the face of the transducer and the surface of the block. Adjust this distance accurately, within a tolerance of ±1/32 inch (±0.8 mm), by using a gauge between the block and the transducer.

b.   Adjust the transducer with the manipulator to obtain a maximum indication height from the front surface reflection of the block. This indication assures that the sound beam is perpendicular to the top surface of the block. A maximum number of back surface reflections serves the same purpose.

c.   Move the transducer laterally until the maximum response is received from the flat-bottomed hole. Adjust the instrument gain control until the indication height is 50 percent of the maximum obtainable.

d.   Replace that reference block with each of the other blocks in the set. Repeat steps "b" and "c" for each block and record the indications. Maintain water-path distance of 3 inches (76.2 mm) for each block except if the basic set is being used. A water-path distance of 6 inches (152.4 mm) is required for the block containing an 8/64 inch diameter hole with a sound-path distance of 3 inches (76.2 mm).

e. Plot a "curve" of the recorded indications as in Figure 4-7. In the example shown, the near zone extends from the 1/2 inch (12.7 mm) sound-path distance indication to the 2 inch (50.8 mm) sound-path distance indication. As the sound-path distance increases beyond 2 inches (50.8 mm), the indications attenuate, or decrease, in height.

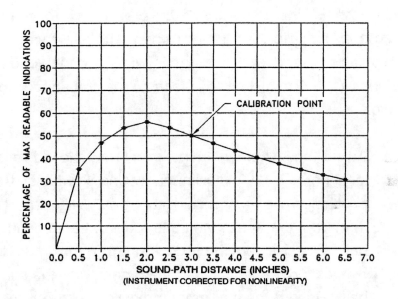

Figure 4-7. Typical Distance Amplitude Response Curve

• Transducer Check

To improve accuracy during test equipment calibration, the characteristics of the transducer, as modified or distorted by the test instrument, may be determined by recording a distance amplitude curve from a 1/2 inch diameter (12.7 mm) steel ball immersed in water. A beam pattern or plot can also be obtained from the same steel ball at a fixed water distance of 3 inches (76.2 mm). It is well to remember that the curve and beam plot recorded in this procedure are not valid if the transducer is subsequently used with

4-15

any test instrument other than the one used in this procedure. A complete analysis of transducer characteristics cannot be accomplished with the commercial ultrasonic testing equipment used in this procedure. To ensure maximum accuracy, the transducer may be calibrated with special equipment. This information is outlined in Chapter 5: Calibrating Transducers. In the procedure that follows, the apparatus used for checking the transducer is the same as that prescribed in the previous paragraphs for calibrating the instrument with reference blocks. The manipulator is set to allow a range in water distance of 0 to at least 6 inches (152.4 mm) from the face of the transducer to the ball surface.

a.   Adjust the instrument gain control until the indication height is 50 percent of the maximum obtainable with the transducer positioned at a water-path distance of $3\pm1/32$ inch (76.2 ± 0.8 mm) from the face of the transducer to the top surface of the ball. Exercise care in producing a true maximum indication by locating the transducer beam center on the center of the ball. Record the maximum indication. Do not readjust the instrument gain control in this or succeeding steps of the procedure.

b.   Vary the water-path distance in 1/8 inch increments through a range of 1/4 inch (6.4 mm) to 6 inches (152.4 mm). Record the maximum indication for each increment of water distance, using care each time the transducer is moved back that the beam center remains centered on the ball.

c.   As in Figure 4-8, plot the recorded indications (corrected for any non-linearity) on a graph to demonstrate the axial distance amplitude response of the transducer and particular test instrument used in the test. The curve for an acceptable transducer is similar to the curve illustrated in Figure 4-11. It is important that the peaks in the curve occur at water distances of 1-1/4, 1-3/4 and 3 inches (31.8, 44.5, 76.2 mm) as shown. The allowable deviation in water distance for the occurrence of these peaks is 1/16 inch (1.6 mm).

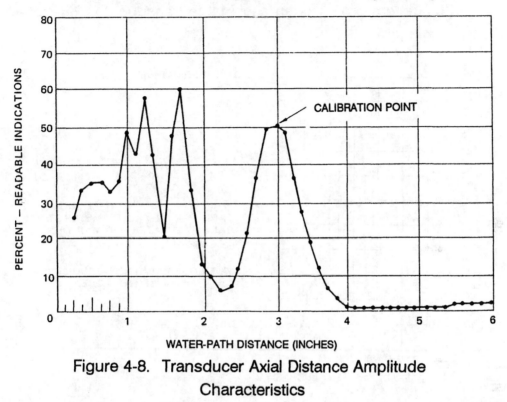

Figure 4-8. Transducer Axial Distance Amplitude Characteristics

d.   Determine the transducer beam pattern by relocating the manipulator to obtain a 3±1/32 inch (76.2±0.8 mm) water-path distance from the 1/2 inch diameter (12.7 mm) steel ball to the face of the transducer. While scanning laterally, 3/8 inch (9.5 mm) total travel, the height of the indication from the ball is observed while the transducer passes over the ball. Three distinct lobes or maximums are observed. The symmetry of the beam is checked by making four scans and displacing each scan by rotating the transducer in its mounting 45°. The magnitude of the side lobes should not vary more than 10 percent about the entire perimeter of the sound beam. Generally, an acceptable transducer would produce a symmetrical beam profile which has side lobes with magnitudes no less than 20 percent nor more than 30 percent of the magnitude of the center lobe. The beam pattern or plot of an acceptable transducer is illustrated in Figure 4-9.

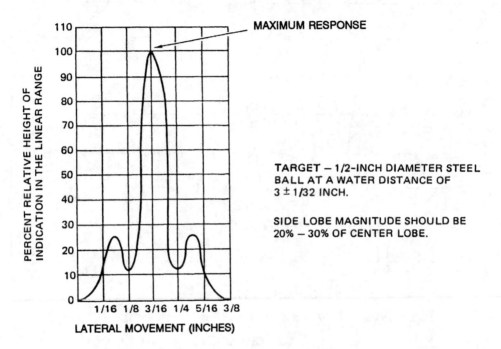

Figure 4-9. Transducer Beam Pattern

Preparation for Testing

● General

Ultrasonic test preparations begin with an examination of the test specimen to determine the appropriate technique. Components are then selected from available equipment to perform the test. Many variables affect the choice of technique. For example, the test specimen may be too large to fit in the immersion tank. In the case of large, fixed structures, the testing unit is moved to the test site. This may require portable testing equipment. Other factors are the number of parts to be tested, the nature of the test material, test surface roughness, methods of joining (welded, bonded, riveted, etc.), and the shape of the specimen. If the testing program covers a large number of identical parts and a permanent test record is desirable, an immersion technique with automatic scanning and recording may be suitable. One-of-a-kind or odd-lot jobs may be tested with portable contact testing units. Each case will require some study as to the most practical and efficient technique.

When setting up any test, an operating frequency is selected, a transducer is chosen, and a reference standard is established. The test specimen is carefully studied to determine its most common or probable discontinuities. For example, in forgings, laminar discontinuities are found parallel to the forging flow lines. Discontinuities (i.e., laminations) in plate are usually parallel to the plate surface and elongated in the rolling direction. Whenever possible, a mockup is manufactured to implant real flaws at critical locations in a specimen to replicate the intended inspection.

● Frequency Selection

High test frequencies are an advantage in immersion testing. In contact testing, 10 MHz is usually the maximum frequency. Low frequencies permit penetration of ultrasound to a greater depth in the material, but may cause a loss of near surface resolution and sensitivity. A sample test specimen is used to evaluate ultrasound penetration with a high-frequency transducer (10 to 25 MHz for immersion and 5 to 10 MHz for contact) and to observe the total number of back reflections. If there is no back surface indication, a lower frequency is required. Successively lower frequencies are applied until several back surface reflections are obtained. If near surface resolution is required, it may be necessary to turn the part over and retest from the opposite side, or to use a high-frequency search unit following the low-frequency scan.

- Transducer Selection

Transducer selection is largely governed by the optimum frequency, as determined in the previous paragraph.

In immersion testing, other considerations include the possibility of using a paintbrush transducer for high-speed scanning to detect gross discontinuities or the possibility of using a focused transducer for greater sensitivity in detecting small discontinuities in near surface areas (no deeper than 2 inches or 50.8 mm). Note that with a given transducer diameter, beam spread decreases as the frequency increases. For example, of two 3/8 inch diameter (9.5 mm) transducers, one 10 MHz and the other 15 MHz frequency, the 15 MHz unit has less beam spread. In contact testing, angle beam units are used for testing welds and relatively thin material.

- Reference Standards

Commercial ultrasonic reference standards have been previously described. These standards are adequate for many test situations, provided the acoustic properties are matched (or nearly matched) between the test specimen and the reference standard. In most cases, responses from discontinuities in the test specimen are likely to differ from the indications received from the reflector in the standard. For this reason, a sample test specimen is sectioned, subjected to metallurgical analysis, and studied to determine the nature of the material and its probable discontinuities. In some cases, artificial discontinuities in the form of holes or notches are introduced into the sample to serve as a basis for comparison with discontinuities found in specimens. For critical applications, a mockup can be manufactured to implant real flaws (cracks, slag inclusions, porosity, etc.) to replicate the component being examined. The implanted flaws usually have a known size (± 0.040 inch or 1 mm) and are placed at strategic locations in the mockup. The UT operator is then required to distinguish the actual defects from geometric reflectors. From these studies, an acceptance level is determined that establishes the number and magnitude of discontinuities allowed in the component being examined. A sensible testing program is then established by an intelligent application of basic material failure theory.

Interpretation of Test Results

- General

Ultrasonic test indications from subsurface discontinuities within the test specimen can be related or compared to indications from reference reflectors of varying depths or sizes in standard test blocks or mockups. These comparisons are a fairly accurate means of evaluating the size, shape, position, and orientation of discontinuities. These conditions, and the discontinuities themselves, are sometimes the cause of ultrasonic phenomena which are difficult to interpret. This type of difficulty can only be resolved by relating the ultrasonic indications to the probable type of discontinuity with reference to the test conditions. Impedance of the material, surface roughness, surface contour, attenuation, and angle of incidence are all to be considered when evaluating the size and location of an unknown discontinuity. The simplest method is to compare the indication of the discontinuity with indications from a reference standard or mockup similar to the test specimen. The experienced operator also learns to discriminate between the indications of actual defects and false or *nonrelevant* indications, as illustrated in Figure 4-10.

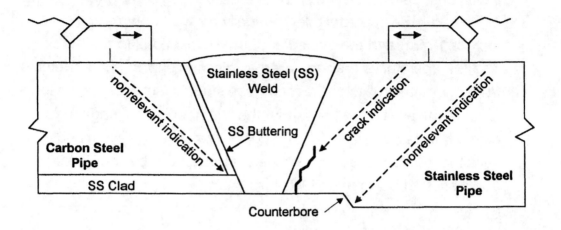

Figure 4-10. Mockup with Nonrelevant Indications

● Typical Immersion Test Indications

Immersion test indications, generally displayed on A-scan pulse-echo units, are interpreted by analysis of three factors: the amplitude of the reflection from a discontinuity, the loss of back surface reflection, and the distance of a discontinuity from the sound entry surface of the article. Individual discontinuities that are small, compared with the transducer's beam spread usually profile the beam (as previously discussed in Transducer Check). Discontinuities larger than the beam spread are evaluated by noting the distance the probe is moved over the test specimen while an indication is maintained. In this case, the amplitude has no quantitative meaning. The length of time the amplitude is maintained does indicate the extent of the discontinuity in one plane. A loss or absence of back surface reflection is evidence that the transmitted sound has been absorbed, refracted, or reflected so that the energy has not returned. Evaluating this loss does not determine the extent of the discontinuity (except when using through-transmission).

When relatively large discontinuities are encountered, the discontinuity may eliminate the back surface reflection, since the sound beam is not transmitted through the discontinuity. Remember though, since the surface of the test specimen and the surface of a discontinuity within it are not as smooth as the surface of the test block and the flat-bottomed hole in the test block, the estimated size of the discontinuity is generally a bit smaller than the actual size.

– Small Discontinuity Indications

A significant number of the discontinuities encountered in ultrasonic testing of wrought aluminum are relatively small. Foreign materials or porosity in the cast ingot are rolled, forged, or extruded into wafer-thin discontinuities during fabrication. The forces used in fabrication tend to orient the flat plane of the discontinuity parallel to the surface of the part. Such a discontinuity and its ultrasonic indication are illustrated in Figure 4-11.

The relationship of the discontinuity indication and its amplitude is determined by comparison with a range of test block flat-bottomed hole reflections as illustrated in Figure 4-12.

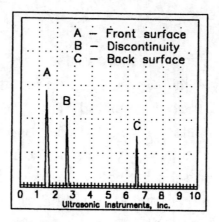

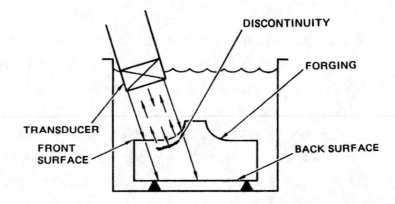

Figure 4-11. Force-Oriented Discontinuity Indication

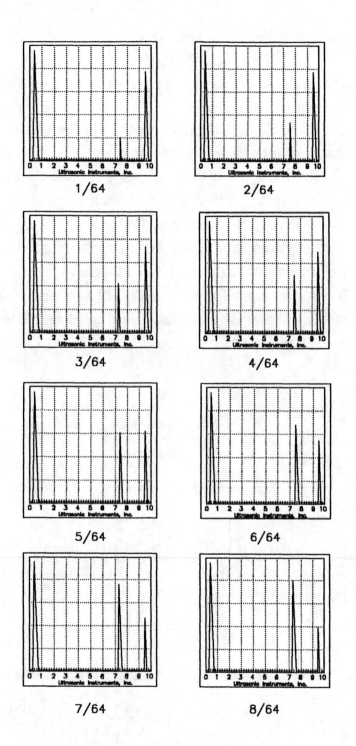

1/64

2/64

3/64

4/64

5/64

6/64

7/64

8/64

Figure 4-12. Amplitude Range of 1/64- to 8/64-Inch Flat-Bottomed Holes

—   Large Discontinuity Indications

Discontinuities that are large, when compared with the beam spread, usually produce a display as in Figure 4-13. Since the discontinuity reflects nearly all of the ultrasound energy, the partial or total loss of back surface reflection is typical. The dimensions of the discontinuity may be determined by measuring the distance that the transducer is moved while still receiving an indication. If the discontinuity is not flat but is three-dimensional, the extent of the third dimension may be determined by turning the article over and scanning from the back side. If the possibility of two discontinuities lying close together is suspected, the article may be tested from all four sides if possible.

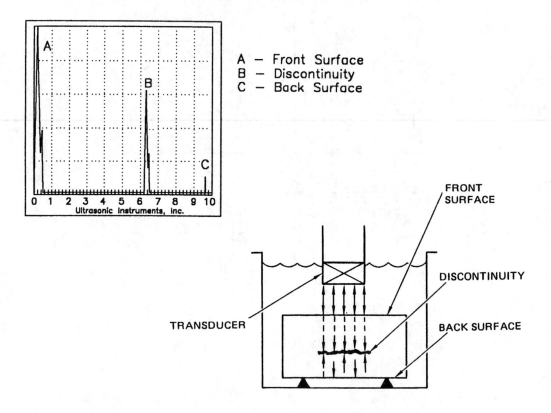

Figure 4-13. Large Discontinuity Indication

— Loss of Back Surface Reflection

Evaluating the loss of back surface reflection is most important when it occurs in the absence of significant individual discontinuities. In this case, among the causes of reduction or loss of back surface reflection are large grain size, porosity, and a dispersion of very fine precipitate particles. Figure 4-14 illustrates the indications received from a sound test specimen and the indications displayed from a porous specimen. Note that the back surface reflections obtained from the porous specimen are reduced considerably.

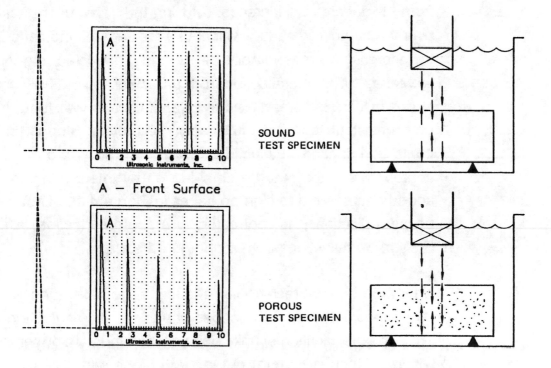

A — Front Surface

SOUND
TEST SPECIMEN

POROUS
TEST SPECIMEN

Figure 4-14. Reduced Back Reflections Due to Porosity

- Nonrelevant Indications

When considering indications that may be nonrelevant, it is a good rule to be suspicious of all indications that are unusually consistent in amplitude and appearance while the transducer is passing over the test specimen. Reflections from fillets and concave surfaces may result in responses appearing between the front and back surfaces. These are sometimes mistaken for reflections from discontinuities. If a suspected indication results from a contoured surface (see Figure 4-15), the amplitude of the indication will diminish as the transducer is moved over the flat area of the front surface. At the same time, the amplitude of the indication from the flat area will increase. Moving the transducer back over the contoured surface will cause the flat area indication to decrease as the amplitude of the suspected signal increases. Where a reflection from an actual discontinuity is strong in localized areas, a nonrelevant indication will tend to be consistent as the transducer is moved along the contoured surface. Reflections which can follow around a contoured surface may be shielded off by interrupting the sound beam with a foreign object as in Figure 4-15. Broad-based indications, as contrasted to a sharp indication, are likely to be reflections from a contoured surface.

Near the edges of rectangular shapes, edge reflections are sometimes observed with no loss of back surface reflection. This type of indication usually occurs when the transducer is within 1/2 inch (12.7 mm) of the edge of the part.

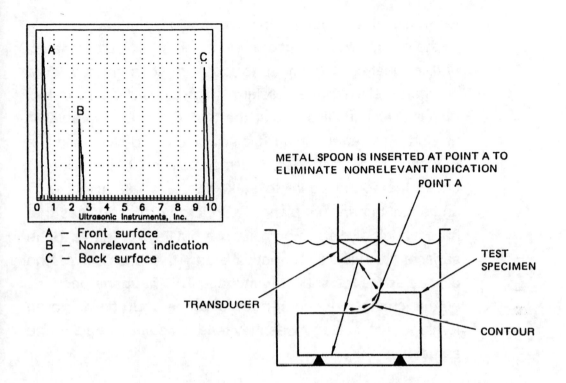

A – Front surface
B – Nonrelevant indication
C – Back surface

Figure 4-15. Nonrelevant Indication from Contoured Surface

Articles with smooth, shiny surfaces will sometimes give rise
to false indications. For example, with a thick aluminum plate
machined to a smooth finish, spurious indications which
appeared to be reflections from a discontinuity located at
about one-third of the article depth were received. As the
transducer was moved over the surface of the plate, the
indication remained relatively uniform in shape and
magnitude. Apparently this type of indication results from
surface waves generated on the extremely smooth surface
and possibly reflected from a nearby edge. They can be
eliminated or minimized by coating the surface with an
ultrasonic couplant.

–   Angled-Plane (Planar) Discontinuity Indications

Discontinuities oriented with their principal plane at an angle to the examination surface are sometimes difficult to detect and evaluate. Usually it is best to scan initially at a comparatively high gain setting (high sensitivity) to detect planar discontinuities. Later the transducer is manipulated around the area of the discontinuity to evaluate its magnitude. In this case, the manipulation is intended to cause the sound beam to strike the discontinuity at right angles to its principal plane. With large discontinuities that have a relatively flat, smooth surface but lie at an angle to the surface, the indication moves along the baseline of the display as the transducer is moved. This happens because of the change in sound-path distance. Bursts in large forgings fit this category as they tend to lie at an angle to the surface.

–   Grain Size Indications

Unusually large grain size in the test specimen may produce "hash" or noise indications as illustrated in Figure 4-16. In the same illustration, note the clearer indications received from the same type of material with fine grain. In some cases, abnormally large grain size results in a total loss of back surface reflection. These conditions are usually brought about by prolonged or improper forging temperatures or high temperature during hot working and subsequent improper annealing of the test specimen. Such multisized grain structures are common in austenitic stainless steel materials and often reduce the signal-to-noise ratio significantly.

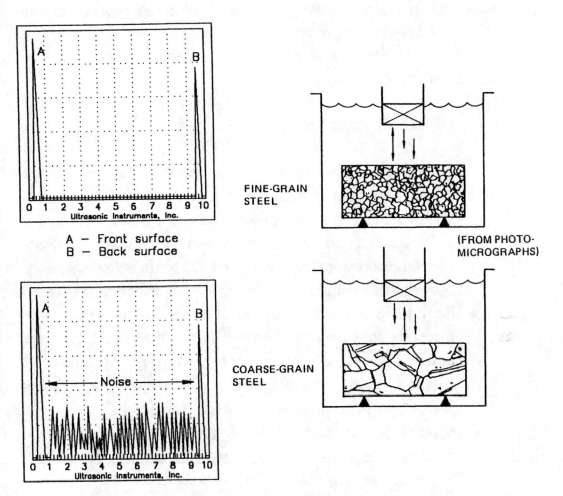

A — Front surface
B — Back surface

FINE-GRAIN STEEL

COARSE-GRAIN STEEL

(FROM PHOTO-MICROGRAPHS)

Figure 4-16. Grain Size Indications

● Typical Contact Test Indications

Contact test indications, in many instances, are similar or identical to those discussed in the previous paragraphs on immersion test indications. Little additional discussion will be given when contact indications are similar to immersion indications. Interference from the initial pulse at the front surface of the test specimen, variations in efficiency of coupling, and poor wedge design in angle beam testing produce nonrelevant effects that are sometimes difficult to recognize in contact testing. As in immersion testing, signal amplitude, loss of back reflection, and distance of the discontinuity from the surfaces of the article are all major factors used in evaluation of the display.

- Dead Zone Indications

  The dead zone is an area directly beneath the front surface from which no reflections are displayed because of obstruction by the initial pulse. In most contact testing, the initial pulse obscures the front surface indication. Near surface discontinuities may be difficult to detect with straight beam transducers because of the initial pulse interference. Shortening the pulse may be effective when near surface discontinuities are obscured by the ringing "tail" of the initial pulse. Figure 4-17 shows a comparison of long and short pulses applied to the test specimen where the discontinuity is near the surface. Only by inserting a standoff, such as a plastic block, or utilizing a dual-element probe can separation of these responses be achieved in contact testing. In immersion testing, the initial pulse is separated from the front surface indication by the water path.

- Typical Discontinuity Indications

  Typical indications encountered in ultrasonic testing include those from discontinuities such as nonmetallic inclusions, seams, forging bursts, cracks, and flaking found in forgings as in Figure 4-18.

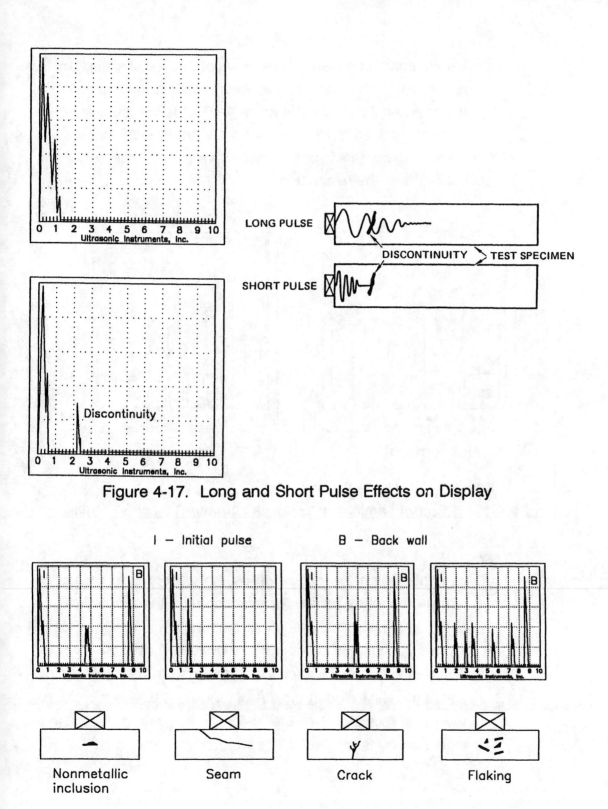

Figure 4-17. Long and Short Pulse Effects on Display

I — Initial pulse   B — Back wall

Nonmetallic   Seam   Crack   Flaking
inclusion

Figure 4-18. Typical Contact Test Discontinuity Indications

Laminations in rolled sheet and plate are defined by a reduction in the distance between back surface reflection multiples as illustrated in Figure 4-19. View A illustrates the display received from a normal plate and View B shows the back surface reflections received when the transducer is moved over the lamination.

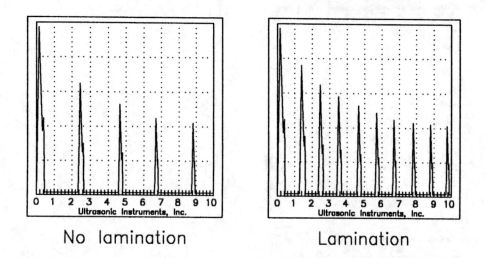

No lamination   Lamination

Figure 4-19. Effect of Lamination on Back Surface Reflection Multiples

In angle beam testing of welds, an acceptable weld area usually responds by lack of indications in the display. Only discontinuities would result in indications. However some of these "discontinuities" may be nonrelevant or metallurgical. Such "metallurgical" indications occurring at the weld fusion zones are illustrated in View A of Figure 4-20. View B shows the same reflections for the fusion zones, but in this case a discontinuity is located in the weld.

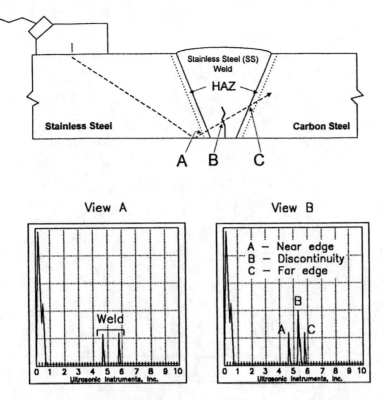

Figure 4-20. Weld Indications Using Angle Beam Contact Techniques

This most often occurs when there are different materials (carbon steel and stainless steel for example) welded together and there are different alloys used in the weldment. The weld itself is essentially a cast material embedded in a mold created by the base metal forming the joint. Therefore, this fusion or heat-affected zone (HAZ) between the base metal being joined and the weld area may cause indications due to reflections of the ultrasound. Depending on the material being joined and the weld filler material, such reflectors may be more pronounced or not present at all. The weld groove commonly has discontinuities such as porosity and slag that produce indications as illustrated in Figure 4-21.

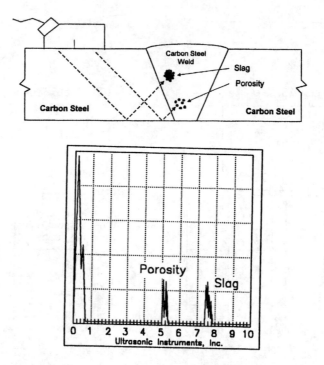

Figure 4-21. Porosity and Slag Indications in Weld Groove

Surface cracks are sometimes detected when testing with a shear wave produced by an angle beam transducer. Figure 4-22 shows a surface wave indication from a crack in the surface of the test specimen.

With pitch-and-catch testing using two transducers, the initial pulse does not interfere with reception as it does when using the single transducer. Figure 4-23 illustrates the indications received from a relatively thin test specimen using two transducers. Tandem or dual angle beam transducers are used to improve near surface resolution. The transit time of the ultrasound when passing through the Lucite wedge on which the transducers are mounted are given an additional advantage in that the initial pulse is moved to the left in the same way the water-path separation occurs in immersion testing. Figure 4-24 shows an indication from a discontinuity which lies only 0.02 inch (0.5 mm) below the sound entry surface of the material.

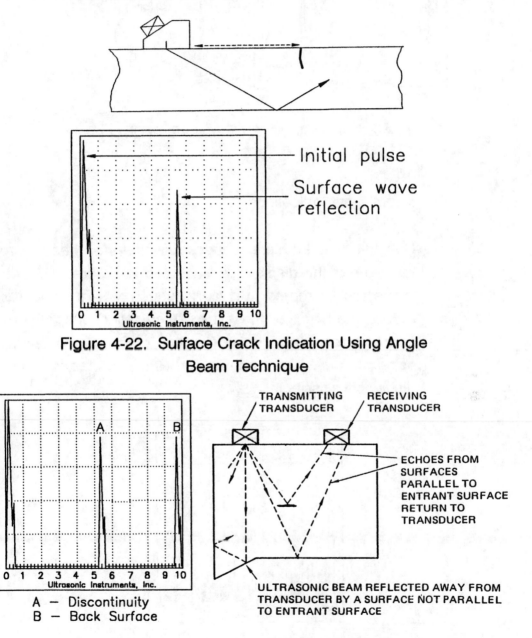

Figure 4-22. Surface Crack Indication Using Angle
Beam Technique

A — Discontinuity
B — Back Surface

Figure 4-23. Two-Transducer Indications

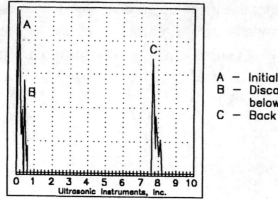

A — Initial pulse
B — Discontinuity 0.02"
    below sound entry surface
C — Back surface

Figure 4-24.   Indications of Near Surface Discontinuity

—   Nonrelevant Indications

Coarse-grained material causes reflections or "hash" across
the width of the display (as illustrated in Figure 4-25) when
the test is attempted at a high frequency.   To eliminate or
reduce the effect of these unwanted reflections, lower the
frequency and change the direction of the sound beam by
using an angle beam transducer with a shorter sound-path
distance if possible.

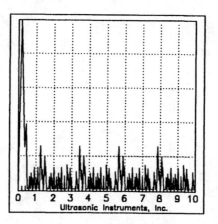

Figure 4-25.   Coarse-Grained Indications

When testing cylindrical specimens (especially when the face of the transducer is not curved to fit the test surface), additional indications following the back surface indication will appear as in Figure 4-26.

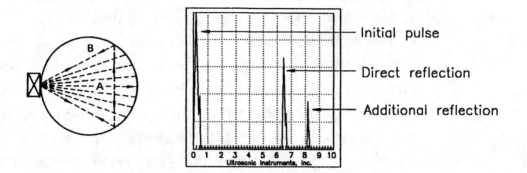

Figure 4-26. Nonrelevant Indication from Cylindrical Specimen

In testing long specimens, mode conversion occurs from the sound beam striking the sides of the test specimen and returning as reflected shear waves as illustrated in Figure 4-27. Changing to a larger diameter (narrower sound beam) transducer will lessen this problem.

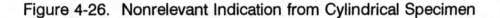
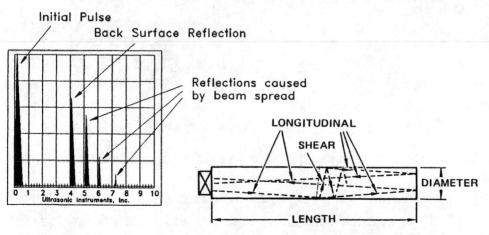

Figure 4-27. Nonrelevant Indication from Long Bar Specimen

Surface waves generated during straight beam testing also cause unwanted nonrelevant indications when they reflect from the edge of the test specimen as in Figure 4-28. This type of nonrelevant indication is easily identified since movement of the transducer will cause the indication from the surface wave to move across the display with the movement of the transducer. When testing with two angle beam transducers, it is possible to have a small surface wave component of the sound beam transmitted to the receiving unit. This type of reflection is readily recognized by varying the distance between the transducers and watching the indication. When the distance is increased, the apparent discontinuity indication moves away from the initial pulse.

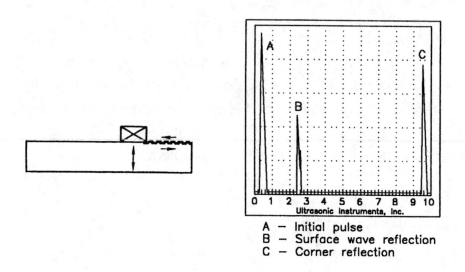

A — Initial pulse
B — Surface wave reflection
C — Corner reflection

Figure 4-28. Nonrelevant Surface Wave Edge Reflection

When using angle beam transducers, a certain amount of unwanted reflections are received from the wedge. These indications appear immediately following the initial pulse as illustrated in Figure 4-29. The reflections from within the wedge are easily identified because they are still present on the display when the transducer is lifted off the test specimen.

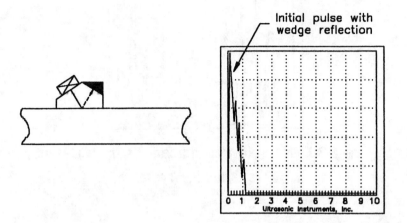

Figure 4-29. Nonrelevant Indication from Plastic Wedge

With continued use, the piezoelectric crystal in the transducer may become defective. When this happens, the indication may be characterized by a prolonged ringing which adds a "tail" to the initial pulse as in Figure 4-30. As the prolonged ringing effect results in a reduced capability of the system to detect discontinuities, the transducer is discarded or repaired.

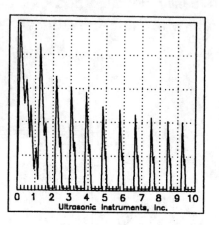

Figure 4-30. Nonrelevant Indications from Defective
Transducer Crystal

Tip Diffraction

● General

"Tip diffraction" is a technique useful for establishing the extremities
of cracks that primarily propagate through the thickness of plates,
pipes, and vessels. The concept is to take advantage of the signal
generated from the tip of the flaw as it diffracts or bends the
ultrasound beam passing over or under it. Notice in Figure 4-31
that the bending of the incident beam results in a wave that
propagates from the top or tip of the notch. This signal locates the
endpoint of the crack and defines its through-wall dimension. Tip
diffracted signals can be generated by either the shear or
longitudinal wave modes.   The use of longitudinal waves
complicates the interpretation, as both longitudinal waves and shear
waves will be present in the test specimen. This testing approach
is known as *bimodal* testing. We will concentrate on contact pulse-
echo approaches of the tip diffraction technique.

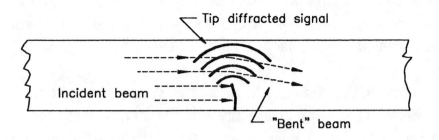

Figure 4-31. Tip Diffraction Concept

A typical application of the technique is in sizing or assessing a crack's height as measured from the inside of the component toward the outside or vice versa. From Figure 4-31 we can see that a signal will be reflected at the base of the crack. Likewise, a tip diffracted signal will be generated at the tip as long as the crack height does not exceed the beam spread. For deeper cracks, we simply move the search unit until we maximize the tip signal; however, characterizing the tip signal in this fashion can be a challenge, even for the most experienced technicians.

Applications of tip diffraction techniques include:

- sizing of under-clad cracking in pressure vessels and piping.
- determination of through-wall dimension of cracks in pipe that has been overlayed with multilayers of weld material.
- determination of the size or diameter of porosity in welds, composites, and ceramics.

Calibration for tip diffraction for through-wall dimensional assessment of inside diameter (ID) connected cracking requires a reference block that contains notches. These notches range from approximately 10 percent to 90 percent through-wall in 5 percent to

10 percent increments. The calibration is done in terms of depth as opposed to sound-path distance. Essentially, as the notch height increases, the time-of-flight for the tip signal decreases; therefore the tip signal arrives earlier in time or closer to the initial pulse.

You realize that the corner trap signal will always peak at the same location in the display, and that is the screen position representing the thickness of the plate or test article. The only indication that will change CRT positions will be the tip signal. It will move closer to the initial pulse as the crack height increases. UT system displays are presented in Figure 4-32 to illustrate the point.

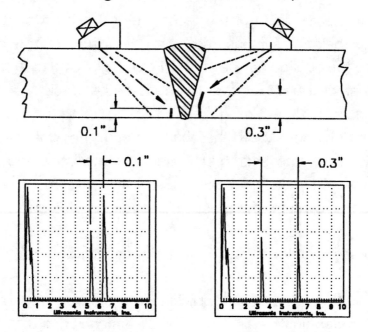

Figure 4-32. Corner Trap and Tip Diffracted Indications

Angle Beam Flaw Locator

It is possible to make a simple, but accurate, "flaw locator" by making a photocopy of the figures on the next few pages. This simple technique will help you understand the concept of angle beam inspection as shown in Figure 4-33. Photocopying Figures 4-34 through 4-39 for individual use is authorized by the publisher. Refer to Appendices E and F for samples of calibration sheets and data recording forms.

With the simple drawing program on your computer, you can generate similar sheets to cover any thickness of material or sound-path angle. Follow these steps when you have access to a calibrated ultrasonic instrument and a specimen with a known flaw.

STEP 1   Obtain maximum UT signal from indication and determine the **surface distance** from exit point of transducer to the weld centerline.

STEP 2   While maintaining the maximum UT signal, determine **sound-path distance** by reading the screen on a properly calibrated UT instrument.

STEP 3   Place transparency on top of the proper sound-path angle (45°, 60° or 70°) and move to match the surface distance in Step 1.

STEP 4   Use a grease pencil to mark the flaw location which will be at the sound-path distance in Step 2.

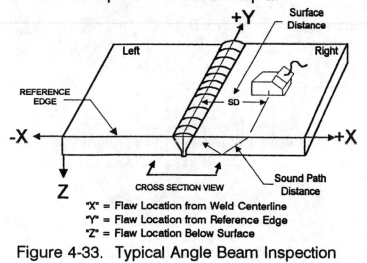

"X" = Flaw Location from Weld Centerline
"Y" = Flaw Location from Reference Edge
"Z" = Flaw Location Below Surface

Figure 4-33. Typical Angle Beam Inspection

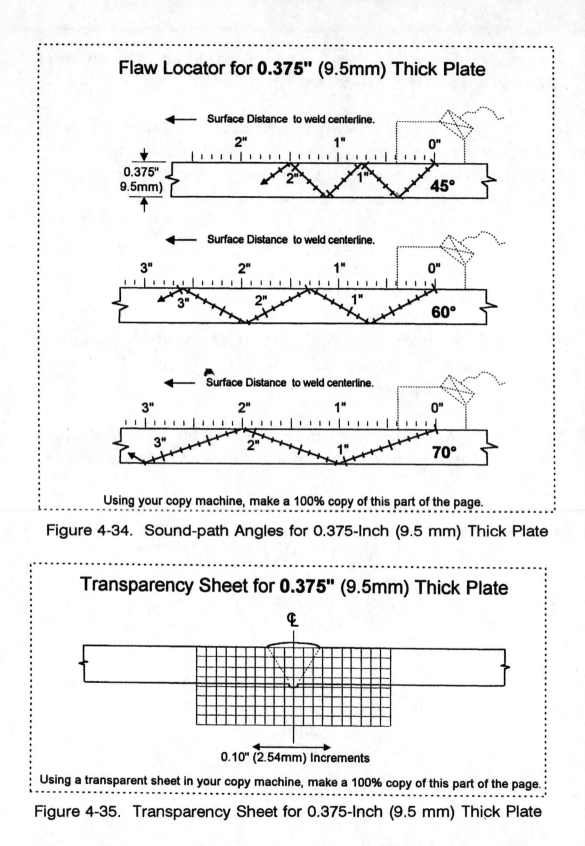

Figure 4-34. Sound-path Angles for 0.375-Inch (9.5 mm) Thick Plate

Figure 4-35. Transparency Sheet for 0.375-Inch (9.5 mm) Thick Plate

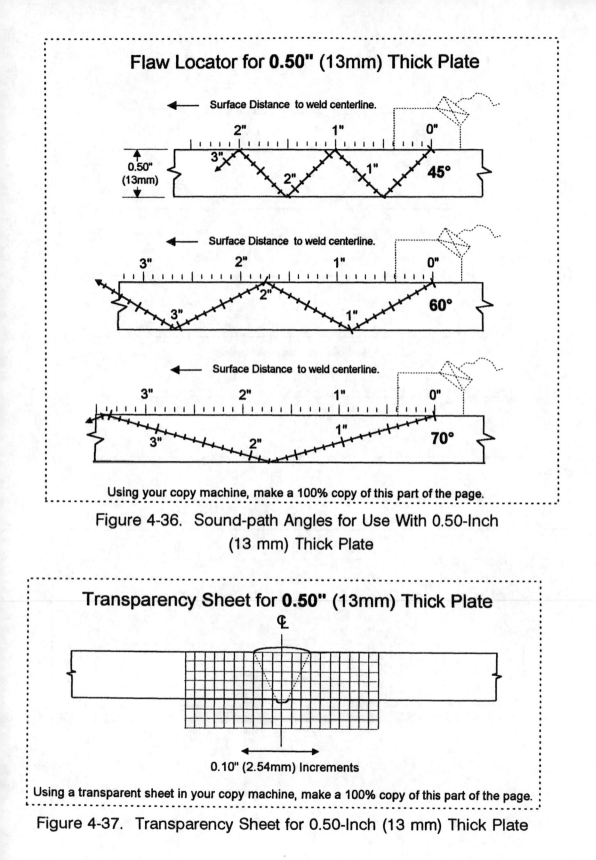

Flaw Locator for **0.50"** (13mm) Thick Plate

Surface Distance to weld centerline.

2" 1" 0"

3"

0.50"
(13mm)

1"

2"

45°

Surface Distance to weld centerline.

3" 2" 1" 0"

2"

3"

1"

60°

Surface Distance to weld centerline.

3" 2" 1" 0"

1"

3" 2"

70°

Using your copy machine, make a 100% copy of this part of the page.

Figure 4-36. Sound-path Angles for Use With 0.50-Inch
(13 mm) Thick Plate

Transparency Sheet for **0.50"** (13mm) Thick Plate

Ȼ

0.10" (2.54mm) Increments

Using a transparent sheet in your copy machine, make a 100% copy of this part of the page.

Figure 4-37. Transparency Sheet for 0.50-Inch (13 mm) Thick Plate

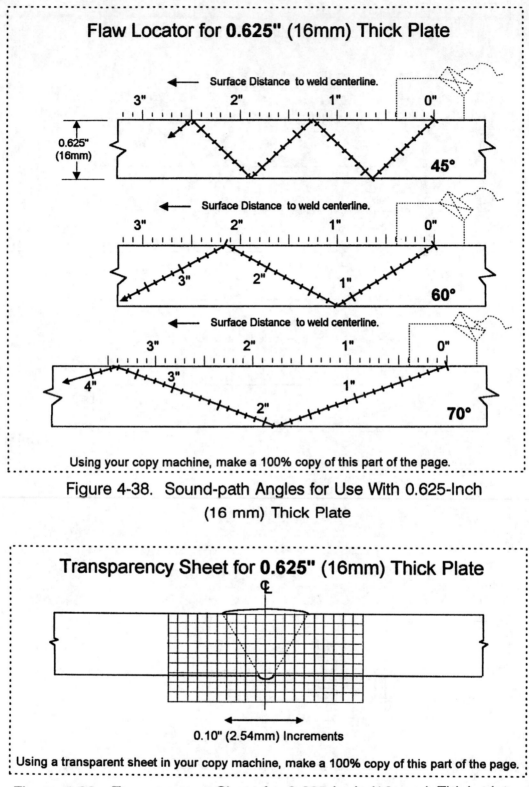

Figure 4-38. Sound-path Angles for Use With 0.625-Inch
(16 mm) Thick Plate

Figure 4-39. Transparency Sheet for 0.625-Inch (16 mm) Thick plate

CHAPTER 5: CALIBRATING TRANSDUCERS

TABLE OF CONTENTS

Page

LIST OF FIGURES

CHAPTER 5

CALIBRATING TRANSDUCERS

General

Ultrasonic transducers, though identical in appearance and manufactured to the same specification, usually have individual characteristics. Acoustic anomalies may exist because of variations in crystal cutting, areas of poor bond to lens, or backing and misalignment of parts in the transducer assembly.

General Equipment Qualifications

Specialized wide-band transmitting and receiving equipment is required to accurately measure transducer variables. Much of these efforts are conducted via computer software programs available from a variety of sources. We will describe the overall process as performed via semi-automated equipment.

In analyzing transducer characteristics, the crystal is excited by a voltage spike that will not distort the natural mode of operation. The return signals received by the transducer are amplified without distortion and are displayed in a manner that will provide a permanent photographic record. The pages that follow describe the special instrumentation equipment and techniques required for measuring or calibrating the recording transducer characteristics such as frequency, sensitivity damping factor, beam size, beam symmetry, and beam focal distance.

General Calibrating Technique

In general, the transducer calibrating technique consists of scanning a small reflector (a ball bearing, a flat post, or a thin wire) in an immersion tank with the ultrasonic beam. As the transducer is moved over the reflector, a changing response that represents a distance amplitude plot of the beam in profile is produced on the oscilloscope. At the highest amplitude portion of the beam, the return signal waveform is photographically recorded while the transducer is held stationary. The waveform is then analyzed to obtain information relating to the frequency, damping ability, and sensitivity of the transducer unit. Using precision manipulative equipment, the transducer is moved over the target and dynamic recording of the beam symmetry is obtained by use of an open-shutter camera. When these recorded measurements are used in specifying or selecting transducers to be used for testing materials or articles, more uniform test results may be expected.

Transducer Calibrating Equipment

- General

  Equipment used to measure the send/receive characteristics of an ultrasonic transducer is capable of reproducing an exact indication on the oscilloscope of the signals sent and received by the transducer. The movement of the transducer over the reflector is accurately controlled. With data potentiometers coupled to sense the motion, a distance amplitude plot of the sound beam is produced on the oscilloscope. An open-shutter camera (or computer programming) is then used to record the beam profile.

- Test Setup

  The transducer is placed in a couplant tank made of Lucite or glass so that the immersed transducer and reflector can be viewed through the couplant. The reflector is scanned by the sound beam with accurate motion of the scanning transducer ensured through the use of milling table crossfeeds to move the transducer. Potentiometers coupled to the crossfeeds convert motion data into electrical signals which are fed into the horizontal position controls. The horizontal oscilloscope display indicates the distance in inches that the transducer traverses. Either X or Y directions of search unit movement are produced by switching from the output of one potentiometer to the output of the other.

- Function

  Figure 5-1 is a functional block diagram of instrumentation equipment. The equipment consists of a timer, a delay unit, a pulser and a wide-band receiver. The unit repeatedly pulses the transducer with a sharp spike and then amplifies the returned signals fed back through the transducer. During operation, the timer triggers both the delay unit and the pulser tube which, at an adjustable time, later triggers the oscilloscope.

- Recording Method

  Figure 5-2 shows how the response curve is recorded (possibly with an open-shutter camera). The sweep delay, as shown, is used to delay the presentation across the oscilloscope screen. By this method, a permanent record, calibrated in thousandths of an inch, (hundredths of a mm) of the response curve describing the uniformity of the sound beam is produced. This information is related to specific abnormalities in the transducer, such as variations in damping, crystal thickness, lens composition, and dimensional nonuniformity.

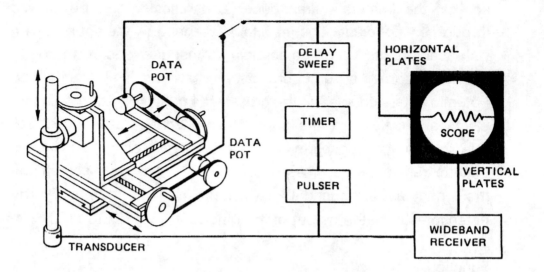

Figure 5-1. Equipment Functional Diagram

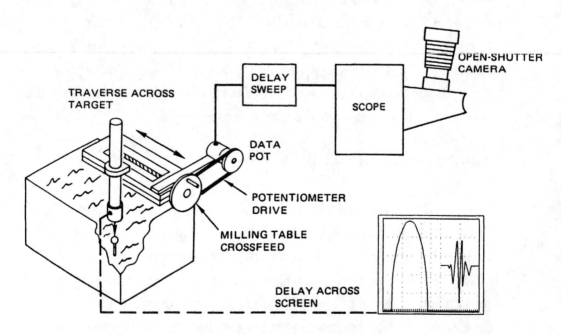

Figure 5-2. Camera Recording Method

- Manipulative Equipment

To obtain precise sound beam and focal length measurements, precision elevating and traversing mechanisms are required. Milling table crossfeeds consisting of heavy micrometer screw slides calibrated in thousandths of an inch (hundredths of a millimeter) are used. Two of the slide screws are fitted with sprocket and chain drives connected to data potentiometers that develop the sweep signal. By relating the micrometer reading to the distance the trace has moved across the oscilloscope screen, the recording is calibrated in inches (or millimeters) per oscilloscope division. The two data potentiometers, one on the transverse and one on the longitudinal movement, are provided so that one plot can be made across the target and then, by switching to the other potentiometer, a plot rotated 90° from the first plot can be made. Thus, two recordings of the beam profile can be made without turning or disturbing the mounting of the transducer.

- Reflector Targets

Reflector targets must be carefully chosen; a bad target will seriously distort the signal and will produce invalid information. In most cases, precision steel balls are used, particularly when calibrating focused transducers. The diameter of the ball must be as small as possible. The size of the effective reflecting surface of the ball is held to less than one-quarter wavelength of the transducer frequency to prevent frequency distortion and undue influence of the target on the measurement of the beam. When analyzing larger-diameter flat transducers, a ball target may not offer adequate return signal amplitude for profile recording. In that case, a flat-topped post as small in diameter as possible is used. The transducer must be held perpendicular to the flat-top surface while testing. Best results are obtained from the use of ball reflectors, since they eliminate the difficulty in holding the transducer normal to the flat surface.

Selection of ultrasonic reflectors varies with the geometry of each crystal and lens. Reflectors must be small compared with the beam size measured. For example, a flat, circular reflector of 12.5 percent of the crystal diameter is adequate for testing flat-disc transducers used to detect fairly large imperfections. Spherically-focused transducers, used to detect very small areas, produce sound beams much smaller than those produced by unfocused transducers; reflector size is small in proportion. In one experiment, performed by the AEC Hanford Laboratories, the sound beam traversed a 0.029-inch-diameter (0.74-mm) ball.

• Pulser

The transducer test requires a pulser with a short pulse capability. To analyze the natural frequency and the damping characteristics of the transducer, the transducer must be excited with a voltage pulse that will not drive the crystal into any abnormal oscillation. This requirement demands that the pulse duration be as short as possible; much less than one period of the natural resonant frequency of the crystal. For analysis of high-frequency (5 to 25 MHz) transducers, the recommended pulse duration is 0.025 microseconds with a rise time of 10 nanoseconds. (A microsecond is one-millionth of a second and a nanosecond is one-billionth of a second.)

• Wide Band Receiver

To prevent the received signal from becoming distorted, a receiver with a wide-band radio frequency amplifier is used. A recommended receiver is one with a bandwidth of 1.5 to 60 MHz, a rise time response of 10 nanoseconds, and a gain of about 40 dB.

- Display System

An effective display system has sufficient bandwidth and rise time to present the information without distortion. Oscilloscopes and computer monitors (through appropriate software) offer combinations of delay and time base expansion features that are desirable for recording transducer beam profiles.

Recording of Transducer Beam Profiles

- General

Transducer data sheets are prepared, as shown in Figure 5-3, for mounting of photographic records and recording of the transducer analysis factors. The following paragraphs describe various methods used to obtain transducer beam profiles.

- Flat-Disc Transducer Measurements

Figure 5-4 shows a beam profile plot of responses picked up by a flat-disc transducer positioned in water over a reflector made from the butt end of a metal drill which was cut and polished flat. The flat end of the drill and the crystal face were held parallel while the transducer scanned over the reflector along the four parallel paths shown. These four beam amplitude profiles (taken with a moving transducer) plus a return signal waveform (taken with a stationary transducer) were recorded on photographs to provide a permanent record of individual transducer characteristics.

TRANSDUCER ACOUSTICAL ANALYSIS

FREQUENCY DAMPING FACTOR, BEAM WIDTH/DIAMETER, FOCAL LENGTH, BEAM SYMMETRY

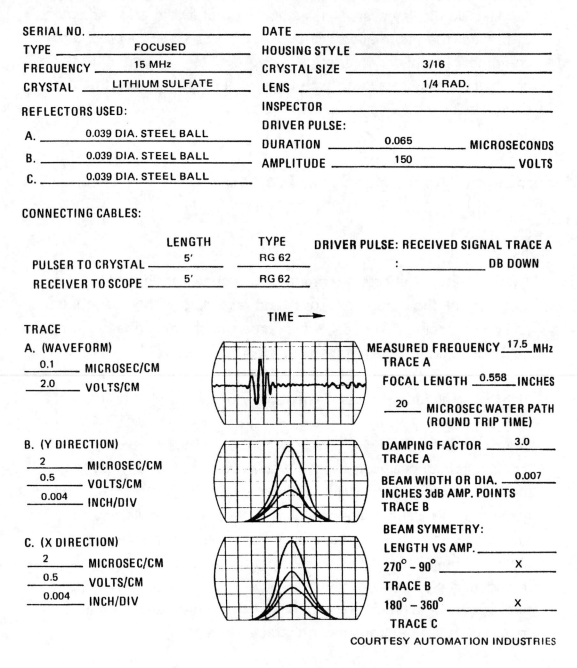

SERIAL NO. _____

TYPE _____ FOCUSED _____

FREQUENCY _____ 15 MHz _____

CRYSTAL ____ LITHIUM SULFATE ____

REFLECTORS USED:

A. _____ 0.039 DIA. STEEL BALL _____

B. _____ 0.039 DIA. STEEL BALL _____

C. _____ 0.039 DIA. STEEL BALL _____

DATE _____

HOUSING STYLE _____

CRYSTAL SIZE _____ 3/16 _____

LENS _____ 1/4 RAD. _____

INSPECTOR _____

DRIVER PULSE:

DURATION ____ 0.065 ____ MICROSECONDS

AMPLITUDE ____ 150 ____ VOLTS

CONNECTING CABLES:

	LENGTH	TYPE
PULSER TO CRYSTAL	5'	RG 62
RECEIVER TO SCOPE	5'	RG 62

DRIVER PULSE: RECEIVED SIGNAL TRACE A

: _____ DB DOWN

TIME ➞

TRACE

A. (WAVEFORM)

____ 0.1 ____ MICROSEC/CM

____ 2.0 ____ VOLTS/CM

MEASURED FREQUENCY 17.5 MHz
TRACE A

FOCAL LENGTH 0.558 INCHES

____ 20 ____ MICROSEC WATER PATH
(ROUND TRIP TIME)

B. (Y DIRECTION)

____ 2 ____ MICROSEC/CM

____ 0.5 ____ VOLTS/CM

____ 0.004 ____ INCH/DIV

DAMPING FACTOR ____ 3.0 ____
TRACE A

BEAM WIDTH OR DIA. ____ 0.007 ____
INCHES 3dB AMP. POINTS
TRACE B

BEAM SYMMETRY:

LENGTH VS AMP. _____

C. (X DIRECTION)

____ 2 ____ MICROSEC/CM

____ 0.5 ____ VOLTS/CM

____ 0.004 ____ INCH/DIV

270° – 90° ____ X ____

TRACE B

180° – 360° ____ X ____

TRACE C

COURTESY AUTOMATION INDUSTRIES

Figure 5-3. Typical Transducer Data Sheet

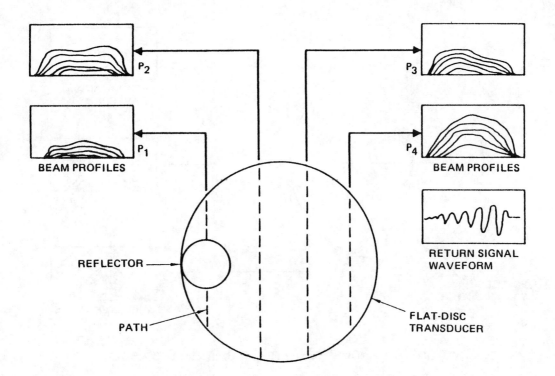

Figure 5-4. Flat-Disc Transducer Measurement

- Focused Transducer Measurements

  Figure 5-5 shows the basic transducer measurements taken from a focused transducer. With the reflector stationary, a waveform was obtained. Two beam amplitude profile plots were taken with the transducer traversed in the X-axis and the Y-axis. If the depth of field for a focused transducer is required, beam profiles may be taken at points inside and outside the focal point.

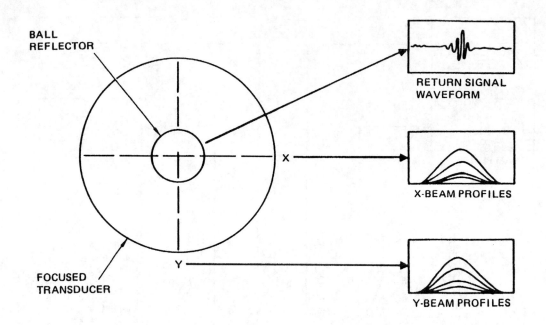

Figure 5-5. Focused Transducer Measurements

- Cylindrically-Focused Transducer Measurements

A wedge-shaped sound beam, focused in width and unfocused along the length, is produced by a cylindrically-focused transducer which has a concave lens. Beam width is measured by traversing the immersed transducer across the length of the beam over a steel ball (or wire) reflector as shown in Figure 5-6. Ball diameter selected depends on the frequency, crystal size and lens radii of the transducer being tested. A rule of thumb is to select as small a reflector as possible that will still produce adequate signal levels for profiling.

Since beam width is usually narrow, the problem of maintaining ball alignment while traversing along the beam length may be avoided by substituting a piece of wire for the ball. The wire diameter depends on the same factors that determine ball diameter selection, i.e., frequency, crystal size, and lens radii.

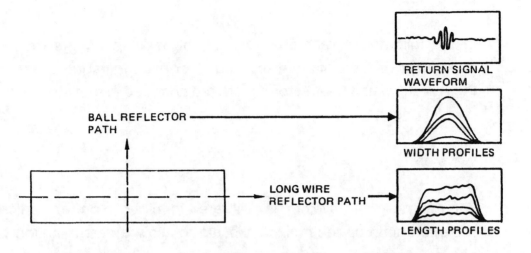

Figure 5-6. Cylindrically-Focused Transducer
Measurements

Two beam amplitude profiles are produced by translating along the beam length over the wire, and then translating across the beam width over the ball reflector.

The point on the reflector selected for the beam width measurement is determined by the position of the transducer when the beam length measurement is at its point of highest amplitude. With the transducer held stationary, the waveform is also recorded at this point. If the depth of field for the focused area of the beam is required, the beam profile is taken with the transducer moved to points where the reflector is nearer than the focal point and beyond the focal point.

Analysis of Transducer Data

- General

    In the following paragraphs each of the main headings on the transducer data sheet are discussed. For each transducer tested, the waveform and beam profile plots are analyzed as outlined in the paragraphs that follow.

- Waveform

    The return signal waveform is calibrated in millivolts on the vertical scale and time on the horizontal scale to allow a determination of crystal frequency, damping factor, and sensitivity.

- Frequency

    In this analysis, the actual frequency of transducer operation is measured and compared to the design frequency. The actual frequency is a measurement of the acoustic wave in the water medium. As this is the frequency of the energy used when testing material, this is the frequency that is recorded. To record the acoustical frequency of the transducer, the first reflected signal from the ball target is analyzed. Trace A in Figure 5-3 illustrates this signal. The frequency may be calculated if the period (time base) is known, since frequency equals the number of complete cycles per unit of time.

- Damping Factor

    The damping factor is defined as the number of positive half-cycles within the pulse that are greater in amplitude than the first half-cycle. By counting the number of cycles generated by the crystal when reacting to the reflected pulse, a measure of the damping factor is reached. Trace A in Figure 5-3 illustrates this measurement. In this method, the damping factor is essentially a measurement of the time required for the crystal to return to a quiescent state after excitation. The resolution of the transducer is directly related to the damping factor. The smaller the damping factor, the better the ability of the transducer to resolve two signals arriving very close together in time.

- Sensitivity

Sensitivity is a measure of the ability of the transducer to detect the minute amount of sound energy reflected from a given size target at a given distance. The vertical amplitude of the signal received, as shown in trace A of Figure 5-3, calibrated in volts per centimeter (unit length) measures sensitivity. With the amplitude and duration of the pulse known and the amplification factor of the wide-band receiver known and held constant, sensitivity is measured in volts peak-to-peak or in decibels down with respect to the pulse voltage. The ultrasonic reflectors used in a test for sensitivity vary with the geometry of the crystal and lens. In general, the reflector is small compared to the beam size measured (roughly equal in size to actual defects the transducer is expected to detect). For flat, straight-beam transducers, a flat, circular reflector of 12.5 percent of the crystal diameter is adequate. Beam sizes of focused transducers, used to detect very small discontinuities, are much smaller than the beam sizes of flat transducers; therefore, the reflector is also smaller. Steel balls ranging in size from 0.030 to 0.050 inch (0.76 to 1.27 mm) in diameter have been used successfully for testing focused units. These tiny balls are also used for measuring the beam width of cylindrically-focused transducers. These units are focused in the width dimension and unfocused along the beam length. If difficulties are experienced in aligning the transducer with the ball while traversing in the beam length direction, a fine, small-diameter wire may be laid along the lengthwise path as a substitute for the ball.

- Focal Length

The focal length information for focused transducers is the water-path distance at which a maximum return signal is obtained. Focal length is the time base measurement on the oscilloscope between the excitation pulse and the point of maximum amplitude response. The transducer is held over the center of the ball target and moved toward or away from the ball until the maximum reflected signal is received. The focal length is then noted and recorded.

- Beam Amplitude Profiles

The beam amplitude profiles show amplitude envelopes of each half-cycle with the vertical scale calibrated in millivolts of transducer return signal and the horizontal scale calibrated in mils, or centimeters, of transducer travel. The motion of the transducer across the target drives a data potentiometer which in turn delays the composite rf (radio frequency) signal across the oscilloscope and a distance amplitude recording for each individual cycle is produced. The highest amplitude cycle records the major envelope, the next highest amplitude cycle records the next lower curve, and so on. This system of recording produces superimposed response curves from each individual cycle with respect to each other. The symmetry of these curves with respect to one another is indicative of uniformity of operation of the transducer in the send/receive modes. The symmetry of these curves is affected by variations in damping, crystal thickness, lens thickness, and bonding of the transducer components.

- Beam Width and Symmetry

The beam width is read directly from the width of the profile envelope displayed on the calibrated horizontal axis, or at the 3 dB down points on each side of the profile peak. Nonsymmetry is recognized as variations in the profile patterns of the propagated sound beam and, through critical analysis of these beam envelope variations, normal and abnormal conditions can be identified. Nonsymmetry may be caused by backing variations, lens centering or misalignment. Porosity in lenses and small imperfections in electrodes and bonding have also been linked to distortion in beam profiles.

APPENDIX A

COMPARISON AND SELECTION OF NDT PROCESSES

TABLE OF CONTENTS

LIST OF FIGURES

APPENDIX A

COMPARISON AND SELECTION OF NDT PROCESSES

General

This appendix summarizes the characteristics of various types of discontinuities and lists the NDT methods that may be employed to detect each type of discontinuity.

The relationship between the various NDT methods and their capabilities and limitations when applied to the detection of a specific discontinuity is shown. Such variables as type of discontinuity (inherent, process, or service), manufacturing processes (heat treating, machining, welding, grinding, or plating), and limitations (metallurgical, structural, or processing) also help in determining the sequence of testing and the ultimate selection of one test method over another.

Method Identification

Figures A-1 through A-5 illustrate five NDT methods. Each illustration shows the three elements involved in all five tests, the different methods in each test category, and tasks that may be accomplished with a specific method.

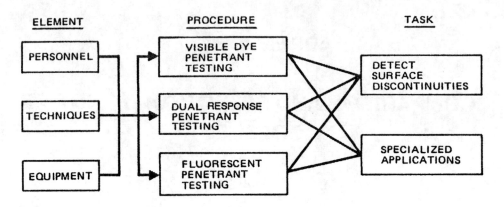

Figure A-1. Liquid Penetrant Test

NDT Discontinuity Selection

The discontinuities that are discussed in the following paragraphs are only some of the many hundreds that are associated with the various materials, processes, and products currently in use.   During the selection of discontinuities for inclusion in this chapter, only those discontinuities which would not be radically changed under different conditions of design, configuration, standards, and environment were chosen.

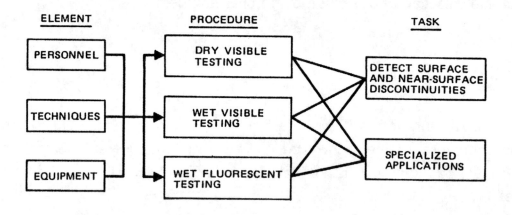

Figure A-2. Magnetic Particle Test

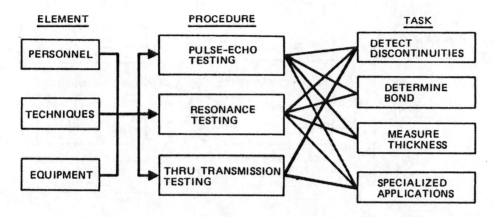

Figure A-3. Ultrasonic Test

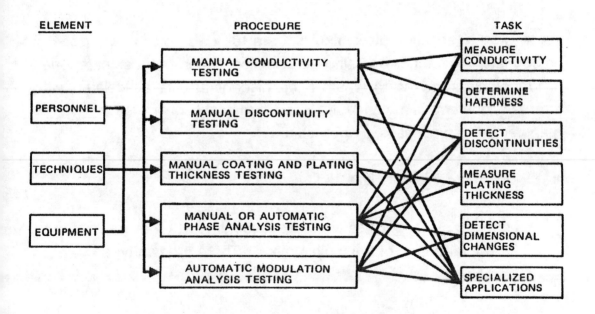

Figure A-4. Eddy Current Test

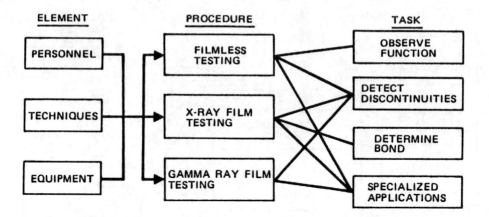

Figure A-5. Radiographic Test

Discontinuity Categories

Each of the specific discontinuities are divided into three general categories: inherent, processing, and service. Each of these categories is further classified as to whether the discontinuity is associated with ferrous or nonferrous materials, the specific material configuration, and the manufacturing processes, if applicable.

● Inherent Discontinuities

Inherent discontinuities are those discontinuities that are related to the solidification of the molten metal. There are two types.

– Wrought

Inherent wrought discontinuities cover those discontinuities which are related to the melting and original solidification of the metal or ingot.

– Cast

Inherent cast discontinuities are those discontinuities which are related to the melting, casting, and solidification of the cast article. It includes those discontinuities that would be inherent to manufacturing variables such as inadequate feeding, gating, excessively-high pouring temperature, entrapped gases, handling, and stacking.

- Processing Discontinuities

Processing discontinuities are those discontinuities that are related to the various manufacturing processes such as machining, forming, extruding, rolling, welding, heat treating, and plating.

- Service Discontinuities

Service discontinuities cover those discontinuities that are related to the various service conditions such as stress corrosion, fatigue, and wear.

Discontinuity Characteristics and Metallurgical Analysis

"Discontinuity characteristics," as used in this chapter, encompasses an analysis of specific discontinuities and references actual photos that illustrate examples of the discontinuity. The discussions cover the following.

- Origin and location of discontinuity (surface, near surface, or subsurface)

- Orientation (parallel or normal to the grain)

- Shape (flat, irregularly-shaped, or spiral)

- Photo (micrograph and/or typical overall view of the discontinuity)

- Metallurgical analysis (how the discontinuity is produced and at what stage of manufacture)

NDT Methods Application and Limitations

- General

The technological accomplishments in the field of nondestructive testing have brought test reliability and reproductibility to a point where the design engineer may now selectively zone the specific article. Zoning is based upon the structural application of the end product and takes into consideration the environment as well as the loading characteristics of the article. Such an evaluation in no way reduces the end reliability of the product, but evaluation does reduce needless rejection of material that otherwise would have been acceptable. Keep in mind that the design engineer must design the most economical component(s), both in terms of cost and use of resources, that will meet the requirements of the application.

Just as the structural application within the article varies, the allowable discontinuity size will vary, depending on the configuration and method of manufacture. For example, a die forging that has large masses of material and an extremely thin web section would not require the same level of acceptance over the entire forging. The forging can be zoned for rigid control of areas where the structural loads are higher, and less rigid for areas where the structural loads permit larger discontinuities.

The nondestructive testing specialist must also select the method which will satisfy the design objective of the specific article and not assume that all NDT methods can produce the same reliability for the same type of discontinuity.

- Selection of the NDT Method

In selecting the NDT method for the evaluation of a specific discontinuity, keep in mind that NDT methods may supplement each other and that several NDT methods may be capable of performing the same task. The selection of one method over another is based upon such variables as those listed below.

- Type and origin of discontinuity

- Material manufacturing processes

- Accessibility of article

- Level of acceptability desired

- Equipment available

- Cost

A planned analysis of the task must be made for each article requiring NDT testing.

The NDT methods listed for each discontinuity in the following paragraphs are in order of preference for that particular discontinuity. However, when reviewing the discussions, it should be kept in mind that new techniques in the NDT field may alter the order of test preference. Literature is available from several resources that addresses many of these specialized NDT methods and techniques.

- Limitations

The limitations applicable to the various NDT methods will vary with the applicable standard, the material, and the service environment. Limitations not only affect the NDT method but, in many cases, they also affect the structural reliability of the test article. For these reasons, limitations that are listed for one discontinuity may also be applicable to other discontinuities under slightly different conditions of material or environment. In addition, the many combinations of environment, location, materials, and test capability do not permit mentioning all limitations that may be associated with the problems of locating a specific discontinuity. The intent of this chapter is fulfilled if you are made aware of the many factors that influence the selection of a valid NDT method.

Burst

- Category - Processing

- Material - Ferrous and Nonferrous Wrought Material

- Discontinuity Characteristics

Surface or internal. Straight or irregular cavities varying in size from wide open to very tight. Usually parallel with the grain. Found in wrought material that required forging, rolling, or extruding (Figure A-6).

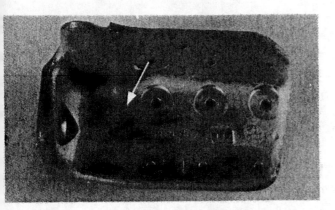

A FORGING EXTERNAL BURST

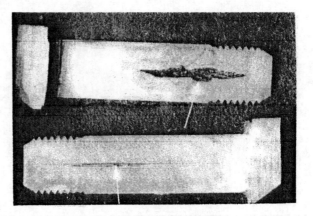

B BOLT INTERNAL BURST

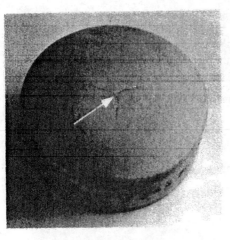

C ROLLED BAR INTERNAL BURST

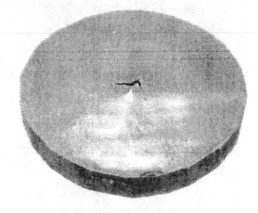

D FORGED BAR INTERNAL BURST

Figure A-6. Burst Discontinuities

- **Metallurgical Analysis**

  - Forging bursts are surface or internal ruptures caused by processing at too low a temperature, excessive working, or metal movement during the forging, rolling, or extruding operation.

  - A burst does not have a spongy appearance and is therefore distinguishable from a pipe, even when it occurs at the center.

  - Bursts are often large and are very seldom healed during subsequent working.

- **NDT Methods Application and Limitations**

  - Ultrasonic Testing Method

    - Normally used for the detection of internal bursts.

    - Bursts are definite breaks in the material and resemble a crack, producing a very sharp reflection on the scope.

    - Ultrasonic testing is capable of detecting varying degrees of burst, a condition not detectable by other NDT methods.

    - Nicks, gouges, raised areas, tool tears, foreign material, or gas bubbles on the article may produce adverse ultrasonic test results.

–   Eddy Current Testing Method

> •   Not normally used. Testing is restricted to wire, rod, and other articles under 0.250 inch (6.35 mm) in diameter.

–   Magnetic Particle Testing Method

> •   Usually used on wrought ferromagnetic material in which the burst is open to the surface or has been exposed to the surface.

> •   Results are limited to surface and near surface evaluation.

–   Liquid Penetrant Testing Method

> •   Not normally used. When fluorescent penetrant is to be applied to an article previously dye penetrant tested, all traces of dye penetrant should first be removed by prolonged cleaning in applicable solvent.

–   Radiographic Testing Method

> •   Not normally used. Such variables as the direction of the burst, close interfaces, wrought material, discontinuity size, and material thickness restrict the capability of radiography.

Cold Shuts

- Category - Inherent

- Material - Ferrous and Nonferrous Cast Material

- Discontinuity Characteristics

Surface and subsurface. Generally appear on the cast surface as smooth indentations which resemble a forging lap (Figure A-7).

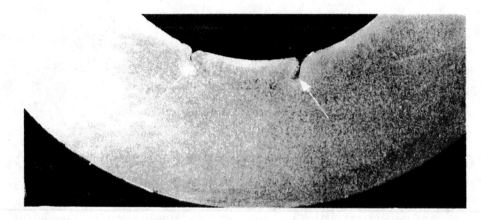

A SURFACE COLD SHUT

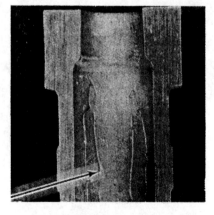

B INTERNAL COLD SHUT

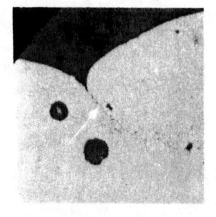

C SURFACE COLD SHUT MICROGRAPH

Figure A-7. Cold Shut Discontinuities

- Metallurgical Analysis

  Cold shuts are produced during casting of molten metal and may be caused by splashing, surging, interrupted pouring, or the meeting of two streams of metal coming from different directions. Cold shuts are also caused by the solidification of one surface before other metal flows over it, the presence of interposing surface films on cold, sluggish metal, or any factor that prevents fusion where two surfaces meet. Cold shuts are more prevalent in castings formed in a mold having several sprues or gates.

- NDT Methods Application and Limitations

  - Liquid Penetrant Testing Method

    - Normally used to evaluate surface cold shuts in both ferrous and nonferrous materials.

    - Indications appear as a smooth, regular, continuous, or intermittent line.

    - Liquid penetrants used to test nickel-based alloys, certain stainless steels, and titanium should not exceed one percent sulfur or chlorine.

    - Certain castings may have surfaces that are blind and from which removal of excess penetrant may be difficult.

    - The geometric configuration (recesses, orifices, and flanges) of a casting may permit buildup of wet developer, thereby masking any detection of a discontinuity.

- Magnetic Particle Testing Method

  - Normally used for the evaluation of ferromagnetic materials.

  - The metallurgical nature of some corrosion-resistant steel is such that, in some cases, magnetic particle testing indications are obtained which do not result from a crack or other harmful discontinuities. These indications arise from a duplex structure within the material, wherein one portion exhibits strong magnetic retentivity and the other does not.

- Radiographic Testing Method

  - Cold shuts are normally detectable by radiography while testing for other casting discontinuities.

  - Cold shuts appear as a distinct, dark line or band of variable length and width and a definite, smooth outline.

  - The casting configuration may have inaccessible areas that can only be tested by radiography.

- Ultrasonic Testing Method

  - Not recommended. As a general rule, cast structure and article configuration do not lend themselves to ultrasonic testing.

–   Eddy Current Testing Method

  •   Article configuration and inherent material variables require the use of specialized probes.

Fillet Cracks (Bolts)

- Category - Service

- Material - Ferrous and Nonferrous Wrought Material

- Discontinuity Characteristics

Surface. Located at the junction of the fillet with the shank of the bolt and progressing inward (Figure A-8).

- Metallurgical Analysis

Fillet cracks occur where a marked change in diameter occurs, such as at the head-to-shank junction where stress risers are created. During the service life of a bolt, repeated loading takes place whereby the tensile load fluctuates in magnitude due to the operation of the mechanism. These tensile loads can cause fatigue failure starting at the point where the stress risers occur. Fatigue failure, which is surface phenomenon, starts at the surface and propagates inward.

- NDT Methods Application and Limitations

  –   Ultrasonic Testing Method

    •   Used extensively for service-associated discontinuities of this type.

A-15

- A wide selection of transducers and equipment enable on-the-spot evaluation for fillet cracks.

- Since fillet cracks are a definite break in the material, the scope pattern will be a very sharp reflection. (Propagation can be monitored by using ultrasonics.)

- Ultrasonic equipment has extreme sensitivity, and established standards should be used to give reproducible and reliable results.

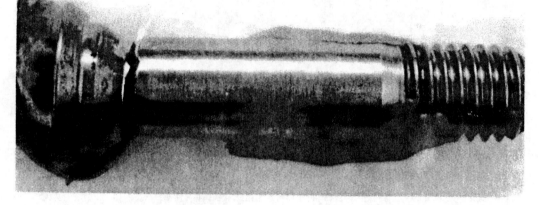

A FILLET FATIGUE FAILURE

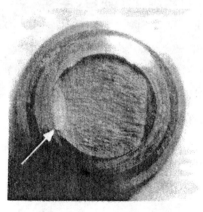 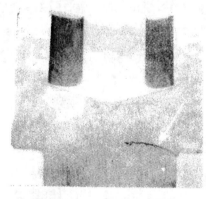

B FRACTURE AREA OF (A) SHOWING TANGENCY POINT OF FAILURE

C CROSS-SECTIONAL AREA OF FATIGUE CRACK IN FILLET SHOWING TANGENCY POINT IN RADIUS

Figure A-8. Fillet Crack Discontinuity

- Liquid Penetrant Testing Method

  • Normally used during inservice overhaul or troubleshooting.

  • May be used for both ferromagnetic and nonferromagnetic bolts, although usually confined to the nonferromagnetic.

  • Fillet cracks appear as sharp, clear indications.

  • Structural damage may result from exposure of high-strength steels to paint strippers, alkaline coating removers, deoxidizer solutions, etc.

  • Entrapment of penetrant under fasteners, in holes, under splices, and in similar areas may cause corrosion due to the penetrant's affinity for moisture.

- Magnetic Particle Testing Method

  • Only used on ferromagnetic bolts.

  • Fillet cracks appear as sharp, clear indications with a heavy buildup.

  • Sharp fillet areas may produce nonrelevant magnetic indications.

  • 16.6 pH steel is only slightly magnetic in the annealed condition; however, it becomes strongly magnetic after heat treatment and can then be magnetic particle tested.

— Eddy Current Testing Method

- Not normally used for detection of fillet cracks. Other NDT methods are more compatible to the detection of this type of discontinuity.

— Radiographic Testing Method

- Not normally used for detection of fillet cracks. Surface discontinuities of this type would be difficult to evaluate due to the size of the crack in relation to the thickness of the material.

Grinding Cracks

- Category - Processing

- Material - Ferrous and Nonferrous

- Discontinuity Characteristics

Surface. Very shallow and sharp at the root. Similar to heat-treat cracks and usually, but not always, occur in groups. Grinding cracks generally occur at right angles to the direction of grinding. They are found in highly heat-treated articles, chrome-plated, case-hardened, and ceramic materials that are subjected to grinding operations (Figure A-9).

- Metallurgical Analysis

Grinding of hardened surfaces frequently introduces cracks. These thermal cracks are caused by local overheating of the surface being ground. The overheating is usually caused by lack of coolant or poor coolant, a dull or improperly ground wheel, too rapid feed or too heavy cut.

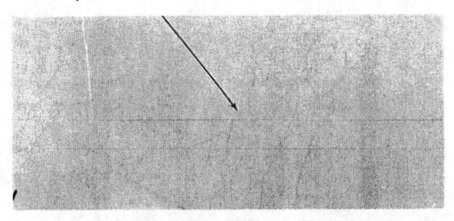

A   TYPICAL CHECKED GRINDING CRACK PATTERN

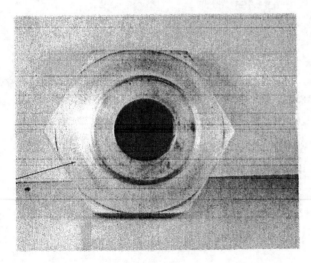

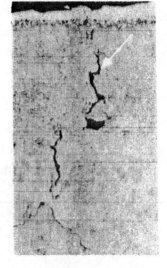

B   GRINDING CRACK PATTERN NORMAL TO GRINDING   C   MICROGRAPH OF GRINDING CRACK

Figure A-9. Grinding Crack Discontinuity

- NDT Methods Application and Limitations

    – Liquid Penetrant Testing Method

A-19

- Normally used on both ferrous and nonferrous materials for the detection of grinding cracks.

- Liquid penetrant indication will appear as an irregular, a checked, or a scattered pattern of fine lines.

- Grinding cracks are the most difficult discontinuities to detect and require the longest penetration time.

- Articles that have been degreased may still have solvent entrapped in the discontinuity and should be allowed sufficient time for evaporation prior to application of the penetrant.

- Magnetic Particle Testing Method

  - Restricted to ferromagnetic materials.

  - Grinding cracks generally occur at right angles to grinding direction, although in extreme cases a complete network of cracks may appear. In this case they may be parallel to the magnetic field.

  - Magnetic sensitivity decreases as the size of the grinding crack decreases.

- Eddy Current Testing Method

  - Although not normally used for detection of grinding cracks, eddy current equipment has the capability and can be developed for specific ferrous and nonferrous applications.

- Ultrasonic Testing Method

  - Not normally used for detection of grinding cracks. Other forms of NDT are more economical, faster, and better adapted to this type of discontinuity than ultrasonics.

- Radiographic Testing Method

  - Not recommended for detection of grinding cracks. Grinding cracks are too tight and too small. Other NDT methods are more suitable for detection of grinding cracks.

Convolution Cracks

- Category - Processing

- Material - Nonferrous

- Discontinuity Characteristics

Surface. Range in size from microfractures to open fissures. Situated on the periphery of the convolutions and extend longitudinally in direction of rolling (Figure A-10).

- Metallurgical Analysis

A rough "orange peel" effect of convolution cracks is the result of either a forming operation that stretches the material or from chemical attack, such as pickling treatment. The roughened surface contains small pits that form stress risers. Subsequent service application (vibration and flexing) may introduce stresses that act on these pits and form fatigue cracks as shown in Figure A-10.

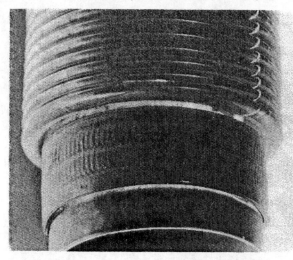

A   TYPICAL CONVOLUTION DUCTING

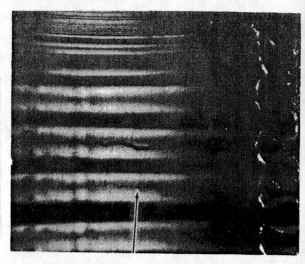

B   CROSS-SECTION OF CRACKED CONVOLUTION

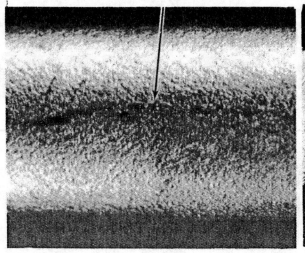

C   HIGHER MAGNIFICATION OF CRACK SHOWING
    ORANGE PEEL

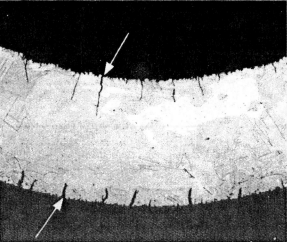

D   MICROGRAPH OF CONVOLUTION WITH PARTIAL
    CRACKING ON SIDES

Figure A-10.   Convolution Crack Discontinuities

- NDT Methods Application and Limitations

  - Radiographic Testing Method

A-22

- Used extensively for this type of failure.

- The configuration of the article and the location of the discontinuity limits detection almost exclusively to radiography.

- Orientation of convolutions to X-ray source is very critical since those discontinuities that are not normal to X-ray may not register on the film due to the small change in density.

- Liquid penetrant and magnetic particle testing may supplement, but not replace, radiographic and ultrasonic testing.

- The type of marking material (e.g., grease pencil on titanium) used to identify the area of discontinuities may affect the structure of the article.

- Ultrasonic Testing Method

  - Not normally used for the detection of convolution cracks. The configuration of the article (double-walled convolutions) and the presence of internal micro fractures are all factors that restrict the use of ultrasonics.

- Eddy Current Testing Method

  - Not normally used for the detection of convolution cracks. As in the case of ultrasonic testing, the configuration does not lend itself to this method of testing.

- Liquid Penetrant Testing Method

  • Not recommended for the detection of convolution cracks. Although the discontinuities are surface, they are internal and are superimposed over an exterior shell, which creates a serious problem of entrapment.

- Magnetic Particle Testing Method

  • Not applicable. Material is nonferrous.

Heat-Affected Zone Cracking

• Category - Processing (Weldments)

• Material - Ferrous and Nonferrous

• Discontinuity Characteristics

Surface. Often quite deep and very tight. Usually run parallel with the weld in the heat-affected zone of the weldment (Figure A-11).

• Metallurgical Analysis

Hot cracking or heat-affected zones of weldments increases in severity with increasing carbon content. Steels that contain more than 0.30 percent carbon are prone to this type of failure and require preheating prior to welding.

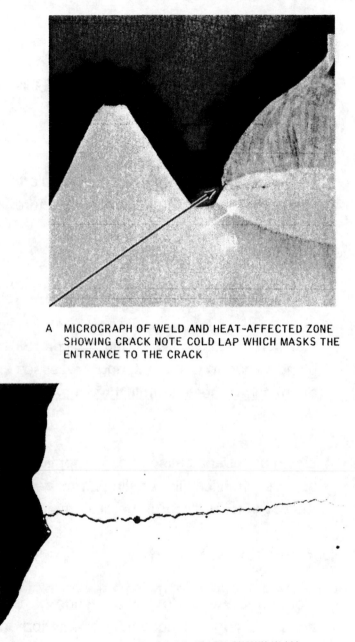

A   MICROGRAPH OF WELD AND HEAT-AFFECTED ZONE
     SHOWING CRACK NOTE COLD LAP WHICH MASKS THE
     ENTRANCE TO THE CRACK

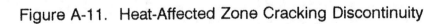

B   MICROGRAPH OF CRACK SHOWN IN (A)

Figure A-11.   Heat-Affected Zone Cracking Discontinuity

- **NDT Methods Application and Limitations**

  - Magnetic Particle Testing Method

    - Normally used for ferromagnetic weldments.

    - Prod burns are very detrimental, especially on highly-heat-treated articles. Burns may contribute to structural failure of article.

    - Demagnetization of highly-heat-treated articles can be very difficult due to metallurgical structure.

  - Liquid Penetrant Testing Method

    - Normally used for nonferrous weldments.

    - Material that has had its surface obliterated, blurred, or blended due to manufacturing processes should not be penetrant tested until the smeared surface has been removed.

    - Liquid penetrant testing after the application of certain types of chemical film coatings may be invalid due to the covering or filling of the discontinuities.

  - Radiographic Testing Method

    - Not normally used for the detection of heat-affected-zone cracking. Discontinuity orientation and surface origin make other NDT methods more suitable.

- Ultrasonic Testing Method

  - Used where specialized applications have been developed.

  - Rigid standards and procedures are required to develop valid tests.

  - The configuration of the surface roughness (i.e., sharp versus rounded root radii and the slope condition) is a major factor in deflecting the sound beam.

- Eddy Current Testing Method

  - Although not normally used for the detection of heat-affected-zone cracking, eddy current testing equipment has the capability of detecting ferrous and nonferrous surface discontinuities.

Heat-Treat Cracks

- Category - Processing

- Material - Ferrous and Nonferrous Wrought and Cast Material

- Discontinuity Characteristics

Surface. Usually deep and forked. Seldom follow a definite pattern and can be in any direction on the part. Originate in areas with rapid change of material thickness, sharp machining marks, fillets, nicks, and discontinuities that have been exposed to the surface of the material (Figure A-12).

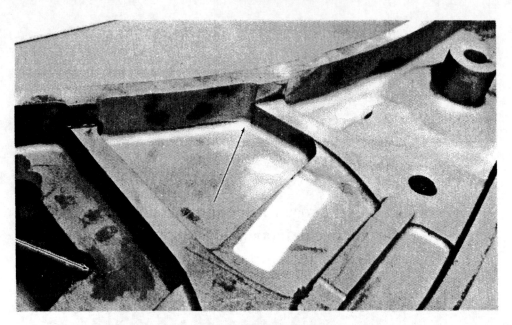

A FILLET AND MATERIAL THICKNESS CRACKS (TOP CENTER)
RELIEF RADIUS CRACKING (LOWER LEFT)

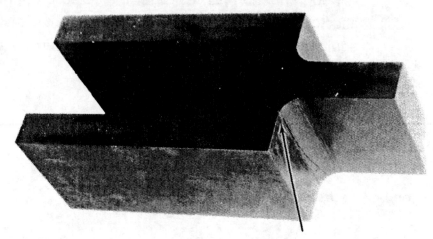

B HEAT-TREAT CRACK DUE TO SHARP MACHINING MARKS

Figure A-12. Heat-Treat Crack Discontinuities

● Metallurgical Analysis

During the heating and cooling process, localized stresses may be
set up by unequal heating or cooling, restricted movement of the

article or unequal cross-sectional thickness. These stresses may exceed the tensile strength of the material, causing it to rupture. Where built-in stress risers occur (keyways or grooves), additional cracks may develop.

- NDT Methods Application and Limitations

  - Magnetic Particle Testing Method

    - For ferromagnetic materials, heat-treat cracks are normally detected by magnetic particle testing.

    - Indications normally appear as straight, forked, or curved indications.

    - Likely points of origin are areas that would develop stress risers, such as keyways, fillets, or areas with rapid changes in material thickness.

    - Metallurgical structure of age-hardenable and heat-treatable stainless steels may produce nonrelevant indications.

  - Liquid Penetrant Testing Method

    - Liquid penetrant testing is the recommended method for nonferrous materials.

    - Likely points of origin for heat-treat cracks are the same as those listed for magnetic particle testing.

- Materials or articles that will eventually be used in LOX systems must be tested with LOX-compatible penetrants.

- Eddy Current Testing Method

  - Although not normally used for the detection of heat-treat cracks, eddy current testing equipment has the capability of detecting ferrous and nonferrous surface discontinuities.

- Ultrasonic Testing Method

  - Not normally used for detection of heat-treat cracks. If used, the scope pattern will show a definite indication of a discontinuity. Recommended wave mode would be surface.

- Radiographic Testing Method

  - Not normally used for detection of heat-treat cracks. Surface discontinuities are more easily detected by other NDT methods designed for surface application.

Surface Shrink Cracks

- Category - Processing (Welding)

- Material - Ferrous and Nonferrous

● Discontinuity Characteristics

Surface. Situated on the face of the weld, fusion zone and base metal. Range in size from very small, tight and shallow to open and deep. Cracks may run parallel or transverse to the direction of welding (Figure A-13).

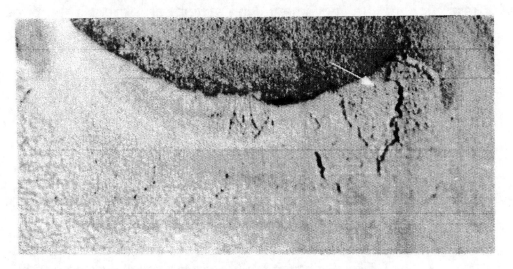

A   TRANSVERSE CRACKS IN HEAT-AFFECTED ZONE

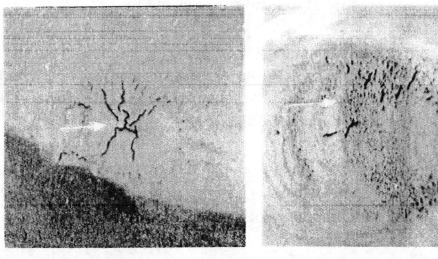

B   TYPICAL STAR-SHAPED CRATER CRACK   C   SHRINKAGE CRACK AT WELD TERMINAL

Figure A-13. Surface Shrink Crack Discontinuities

- **Metallurgical Analysis**

  Surface shrink cracks are generally the result of improper heat application either in heating or welding of the article. Heating or cooling in a localized area may set up stresses that exceed the tensile strength of the material, causing the material to crack. Restriction of the movement (contraction or expansion) of the material during heating, cooling, or welding may also set up excessive stresses.

- **NDT Methods Application and Limitations**

  - Liquid Penetrant Testing Method

    - Surface shrink cracks in nonferrous materials are normally detected by use of liquid penetrants.

    - Liquid penetrant equipment is easily portable and can be used during in-process control for both ferrous and nonferrous weldments.

    - Assemblies that are joined by bolting, riveting, intermittent welding, or press fittings will retain the penetrant, which will seep out after developing and mask the adjoining surfaces.

    - When articles are dried in a hot air dryer or by similar means, excessive drying temperature should be avoided to prevent evaporation of penetrant.

- Magnetic Particle Testing Method

  • Ferromagnetic weldments are normally tested by magnetic particle method.

  • Surface discontinuities that are parallel to the magnetic field will not produce indications, since they do not interrupt or distort the magnetic field.

  • Areas such as grease fittings, bearing races, or other similar items that might be damaged or clogged by the bath or by the particles should be masked before testing.

- Eddy Current Testing Method

  • Ferrous and nonferrous welded sections can be inspected.

  • A probe or encircling coil could be used where article configuration permits.

- Radiographic Testing Method

  • Not normally used for the detection of surface discontinuities. During the radiographic testing of weldments for other types of discontinuities, surface indications may be detected.

- Ultrasonic Testing Method

  • Not normally used for detection of surface shrink cracks. Other forms of NDT (liquid penetrant and magnetic particle) give better results, are more economical, and are faster.

Thread Cracks

● Category - Service

● Material - Ferrous and Nonferrous Wrought Material

● Discontinuity Characteristics

Surface. Cracks are transverse to the grain (transgranular) starting at the root of the thread (Figure A-14).

● Metallurgical Analysis

Fatigue failures of this type are not uncommon. High cyclic stresses resulting from vibration and/or flexing act on the stress risers created by the thread roots to produce cracks. Fatigue cracks may start as fine submicroscopic discontinuities or cracks and propagate in the direction of applied stresses.

● NDT Methods Application and Limitations

  – Liquid Penetrant Testing Method

    • Fluorescent penetrant is recommended over non-fluorescent.

    • Low surface tension solvents, such as gasoline and kerosene, are not recommended cleaners.

- When applying liquid penetrant to components within an assembly or structure, the adjacent areas should be effectively masked to prevent overspraying.

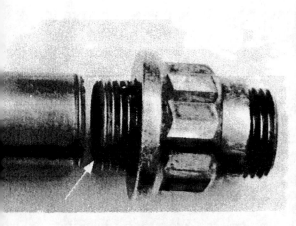

A   COMPLETE THREAD ROOT FAILURE

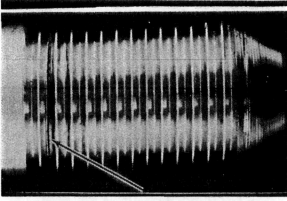

B   TYPICAL THREAD ROOT FAILURE

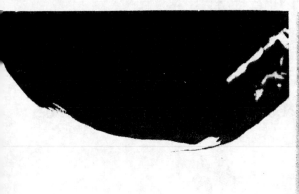

C   MICROGRAPH OF (A) SHOWING CRACK AT BASE OF ROOT

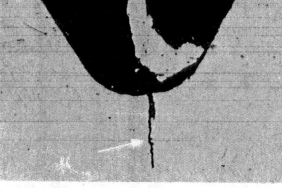

D   MICROGRAPH OF (B) SHOWING TRANSGRANULAR CRACK AT THREAD ROOT

Figure A-14. Thread Crack Discontinuities

- Magnetic Particle Testing Method

    • Normally used to detect cracks at the threads on ferromagnetic materials.

    • Nonrelevant magnetic indications may result from the thread configuration.

    • Cleaning titanium and 440C stainless in halogenated hydrocarbons may result in structural damage to the material.

- Ultrasonic Testing Method

    • The article configuration can be examined utilizing the cylindrical guided-wave techniques. This method requires access to the article and poses interpretation difficulties.

- Eddy Current Testing Method

    • A specialized probe to fit thread size would be required.

- Radiographic Testing Method

    • Not recommended for detecting thread cracks. Surface discontinuities are best screened by NDT method designed for the specific condition. Fatigue cracks of this type are very tight and surface-connected. Detection by radiography would be extremely difficult.

Tubing Cracks

- Category - Inherent

- Material - Nonferrous

- Discontinuity Characteristics

Tubing cracks formed on the inner surface (ID), parallel to direction of grain flow (Figure A-15).

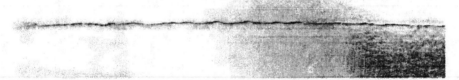

A   TYPICAL CRACK ON INSIDE OF TUBING SHOWING COLD LAP

B   ANOTHER PORTION OF SAME CRACK SHOWING CLEAN FRACTURE

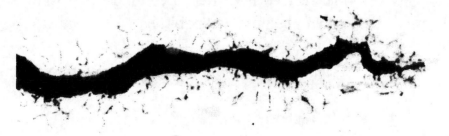

C   MICROGRAPH OF (B)

Figure A-15.   Tubing Crack Discontinuity

- Metallurgical Analysis

  Tubing ID cracks may be attributed to one or a combination of the following:

  - Improper cold reduction of the tube during fabrication.

  - Foreign material may have been embedded on the inner surface of the tubes causing embrittlement and cracking when the cold-worked material was heated during the annealing operation.

  - Insufficient heating rate to the annealing temperature with possible cracking occurring in the 1200°F to 1400°F (649°C to 760°C) range.

- NDT Methods Application and Limitations

  - Eddy Current Testing Method

    - Normally used for detection of this type of discontinuity.

    - Tube diameters below 1 inch (2.54 cm) and wall thicknesses less than 0.150 inch (3.8 mm) are well within equipment capability.

    - Testing of ferromagnetic material may be difficult.

  - Ultrasonic Testing Method

    - Normally used on tubing.

- A wide variety of equipment and transducers are available for screening tubing for internal discontinuities of this type.

- Ultrasonic transducers have varying temperature limitations.

- Certain ultrasonic contact couplants may have high sulfur content which will have an adverse effect on high-nickel alloys.

- Radiographic Testing Method

  - Not normally used for detecting tubing cracks. Discontinuity orientation and thickness of material govern the radiographic sensitivity. Other forms of NDT (eddy current and ultrasonics) are more economical, faster, and more reliable.

- Liquid Penetrant Testing Method

  - Not recommended for detecting tubing cracks. Internal discontinuity would be difficult to process and interpret.

- Magnetic Particle Testing Method

  - Not applicable. Material is nonferrous under normal conditions.

Hydrogen Flake

- Category - Processing

- Material - Ferrous

- Discontinuity Characteristics

Internal fissures in a fractured surface, flakes appear as bright, silvery areas. On an etched surface they appear as short discontinuities. Sometimes known as chrome checks and hairline cracks when revealed by machining. Flakes are extremely thin and generally align parallel with the grain. They are usually found in heavy steel forging, billets, and bars (Figure A-16).

- Metallurgical Analysis

Flakes are internal fissures attributed to stresses produced by localized transformation and decreased solubility of hydrogen during cooling after hot working. Usually found only in heavy alloy steel forgings.

- NDT Methods Application and Limitations

  - Ultrasonic Testing Method

    - Used extensively for the detection of hydrogen flake.

    - Material in the wrought condition can be screened successfully using either the immersion or the contact method. The surface condition will determine the method most suited.

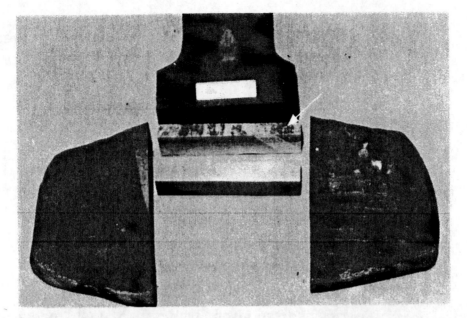

A   4340 CMS HAND FORGING REJECTED FOR HYDROGEN FLAKE

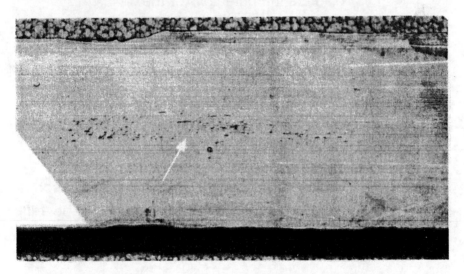

B   CROSS SECTION OF (A) SHOWING FLAKE CONDITION IN CENTER OF MATERIAL

Figure A-16. Hydrogen Flake Discontinuity

- On the A-scan presentation, hydrogen flake will appear as hash on the screen or as loss of back reflection.

- All foreign materials (loose scale, dirt, oil, and grease) should be removed prior to any testing. Surface irregularities such as nicks, gouges, tool marks, and scarfing may cause loss of back reflection.

– Magnetic Particle Testing Method

- Normally used on finish machined articles.

- Flakes appear as short discontinuities and resemble chrome checks or hairline cracks.

- Machined surfaces with deep tool marks may obliterate the detection of the flake.

- Where the general direction of a discontinuity is questionable, it may be necessary to magnetize in two or more directions.

– Liquid Penetrant Testing Method

- Not normally used for detecting flakes. Discontinuities are very small and tight and would be difficult to detect by liquid penetrants.

– Eddy Current Testing Method

- Not recommended for detecting flakes. The metallurgical structure of ferrous materials limits their adaptability to the use of eddy current testing.

- Radiographic Testing Method

  - Not recommended for detecting flakes. The size of the discontinuity and its location and orientation with respect to the material surface restricts the application of radiography.

Hydrogen Embrittlement

- Category - Processing and Service

- Material - Ferrous

- Discontinuity Characteristics

  Surface. Small, nondimensional (interface) with no orientation or direction. Found in highly-heat-treated material that has been subjected to pickling and/or plating or in material exposed to free hydrogen (Figure A-17).

- Metallurgical Analysis

  Operations such as electroplating or pickling and cleaning prior to electroplating generate hydrogen at the surface of the material. This hydrogen penetrates the surface of the material, creating immediate or delayed embrittlement and cracking.

- NDT Methods Application and Limitations

  - Magnetic Particle Testing Method

    - Magnetic indications appear as a fractured pattern.

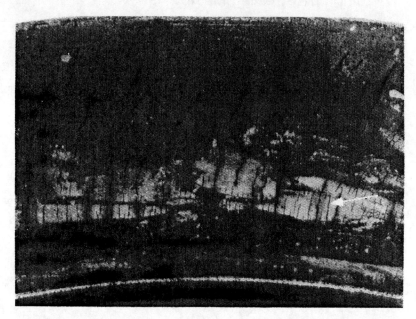

A DETAILED CRACK PATTERN OF HYDROGEN EMBRITTLEMENT

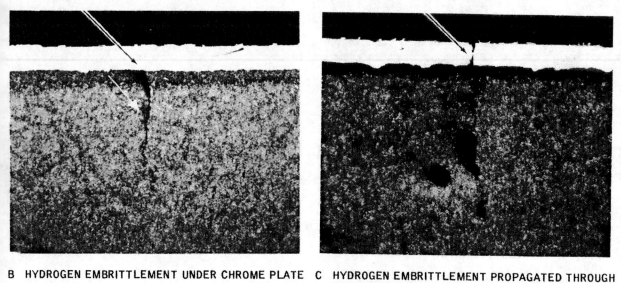

B HYDROGEN EMBRITTLEMENT UNDER CHROME PLATE C HYDROGEN EMBRITTLEMENT PROPAGATED THROUGH
CHROME PLATE

Figure A-17. Hydrogen Embrittlement Discontinuity

- Hydrogen embrittlement cracks are randomly oriented and may be aligned with the magnetic field.

- Magnetic particle testing should be accomplished before and after plating.

- Care should be taken so as not to produce nonrelevant indications or cause damage to the article by overheating.

- Some alloys of corrosion-resistant steel are nonmagnetic in the annealed condition, but become magnetic with cold working.

– Liquid Penetrant Testing Method

- Not normally used for detecting hydrogen embrittlement. Discontinuities on the surface are extremely tight, small, and difficult to detect. Subsequent plating deposit may mask the discontinuity.

– Ultrasonic Testing Method

- Although ultrasonic equipment has the capability of detecting hydrogen embrittlement, this method is not normally used. Article configurations and size do not, in general, lend themselves to this method of testing. Surface wave and/or time-of-flight techniques are recommended.

— Eddy Current Testing Method

- Not recommended for detecting hydrogen embrittlement. Many variables inherent in the specific material may produce conflicting patterns.

— Radiographic Testing Method

- Not recommended for detecting hydrogen embrittlement. The sensitivity required to detect hydrogen embrittlement is, in most cases, in excess of radiographic capabilities.

Inclusions

- Category - Processing (Weldments)

- Material - Ferrous and Nonferrous Welded Material

- Discontinuity Characteristics

Surface and subsurface. Inclusions may be any shape. They may be metallic or nonmetallic and may appear individually or be linearly distributed or scattered throughout the weldment (Figure A-18).

- Metallurgical Analysis

Metallic inclusions are generally particles of metals of different density as compared to the density of the weld or base metal. Nonmetallic inclusions are oxides, sulphides, slag, or other nonmetallic foreign material entrapped in the weld or trapped between the weld metal and the base metal.

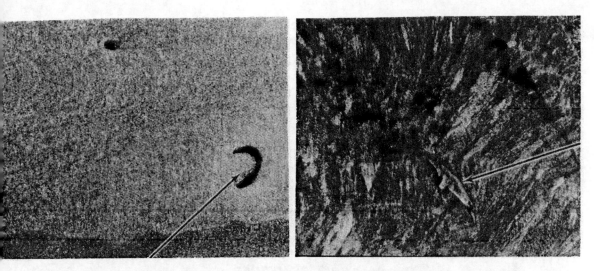

A METALLIC INCLUSIONS   B INCLUSIONS TRAPPED IN WELD

C CROSS SECTION OF WELD SHOWING INTERNAL INCLUSIONS

Figure A-18. Weldment Inclusion Discontinuities

- NDT Methods Application and Limitations

  - Radiographic Testing Method

    - This NDT method is universally used.

    - Metallic inclusions appear on the radiograph as sharply-defined, round, erratically-shaped or elongated white spots and may be isolated or in small linear or scattered groups.

- Nonmetallic inclusions will appear on the radiograph as shadows of round globules or elongated or irregularly-shaped contours occurring individually, linearly or scattered throughout the weldment. They will generally appear in the fusion zone or at the root of the weld. Less absorbent material is indicated by a greater film density and more absorbent materials by a lighter film density.

- Foreign material such as loose scales, splatter, or flux may invalidate test results.

— Eddy Current Testing Method

- Normally confined to thin-walled welded tubing.

- Established standards are required if valid results are to be obtained.

— Magnetic Particle Testing Method

- Normally not used for detecting inclusions in weldments.

- Confined to machined weldments where the discontinuities are surface or near surface.

- The indications would appear jagged, irregularly-shaped, individually, or clustered and would not be too pronounced.

- Discontinuities may go undetected when improper contact exists between the magnetic particles and the surface of the article.

   – Ultrasonic Testing Method

- Not normally used for detecting inclusions. Specific applications of design or of article configuration, however, may require ultrasonic testing.

   – Liquid Penetrant Testing Method

- Not applicable. Inclusions are normally not open fissures.

Inclusions

- Category - Processing

- Material - Ferrous and Nonferrous Wrought Material

- Discontinuity Characteristics

Subsurface (original bar) or surface (after machining). There are two types; one is nonmetallic with long, straight lines parallel to flow lines and quite tightly adherent. They are often short and likely to occur in groups. The other type is nonplastic, appearing as a comparatively large mass not parallel to flow lines. Found in forged, extruded, and rolled material (Figure A-19).

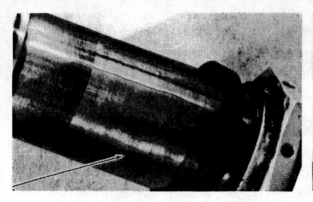

A TYPICAL INCLUSION PATTERN ON MACHINED
   SURFACES

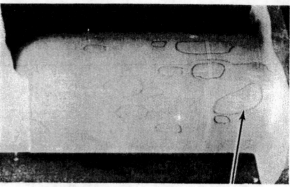

B STEEL FORGING SHOWING NUMEROUS
   INCLUSIONS

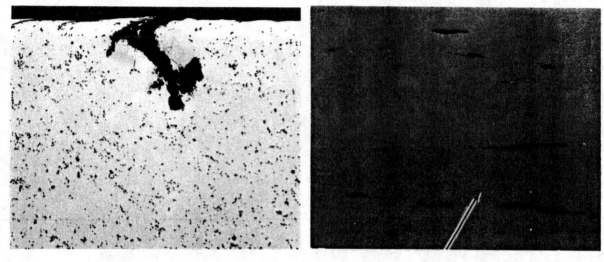

C MICROGRAPH OF TYPICAL INCLUSION

D LONGITUDINAL CROSS SECTION SHOWING
   ORIENTATION OF INCLUSIONS

Figure A-19. Wrought Inclusion Discontinuities

- Metallurgical Analysis

  Nonmetallic inclusions (stringers) are caused by the existence of
  slag or oxides in the billet or ingot. Nonplastic inclusions are
  caused by particles remaining in the solid state during billet melting.
  Certain types of steels are more prone to inclusions than others.

- NDT Methods Application and Limitations

  - Ultrasonic Testing Method

    - Normally used to evaluate inclusions in wrought material.

    - Inclusions will appear as definite interfaces within the metal. Small, clustered condition or conditions on different planes cause a loss in back reflection. Numerous small, scattered conditions cause excessive "noise."

    - Inclusion orientation in relationship to ultrasonic beam is critical.

    - The direction of the ultrasonic beam should be perpendicular to the direction of the grain flow whenever possible.

  - Eddy Current Testing Method

    - Normally used for thin-walled tubing and small-diameter rods.

    - Eddy current testing of ferromagnetic materials can be difficult.

  - Magnetic Particle Testing Method

    - Normally used on machined surface.

- Inclusions will appear as a straight, intermittent, or a continuous indication. They may be individual or clustered.

- The magnetizing technique should be such that a surface or near surface inclusion can be satisfactorily detected when its axis is in any direction.

- A knowledge of the grain flow of the material is critical since inclusions will be parallel to that direction.

– Liquid Penetrant Testing Method

- Not normally used for detecting inclusions in wrought material. Inclusions are generally not openings in the material surface.

– Radiographic Testing Method

- Not recommended. NDT methods designed for surface testing are more suitable for detecting surface inclusions.

Lack of Penetration

- Category - Processing

- Material - Ferrous and Nonferrous Weldments

- Discontinuity Characteristics

  Internal or external. Generally irregular and filamentary occurring at the root and running parallel with the weld (Figure A-20).

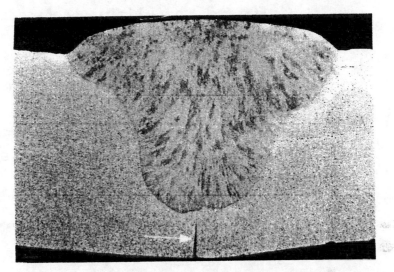

A INADEQUATE ROOT PENETRATION

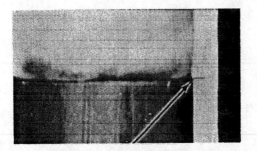

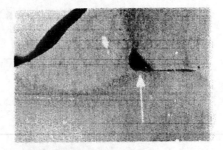

B INADEQUATE ROOT PENETRATION OF BUTT
   WELDED TUBE

C INADEQUATE FILLET WELD PENETRATION
   KNOWN AS BRIDGING

Figure A-20. Lack of Penetration Discontinuities

- Metallurgical Analysis

  Caused by root face of joint not reaching fusion temperature before weld metal was deposited. Also caused by fast welding rate, too large a welding rod or too cold a bead.

- NDT Methods Application and Limitations

  - Radiographic Testing Method

    - Used extensively on a wide variety of welded articles to determine the lack of penetration.

    - Lack of penetration will appear on the radiograph as an elongated, dark area of varying length and width. Lack of penetration may be continuous or intermittent and may appear in the center of the weld at the junction of multipass beads.

    - Lack of penetration orientation in relationship to the radiographic source is critical.

    - Sensitivity levels govern the capability to detect small or tight discontinuities.

  - Ultrasonic Testing Method

    - Commonly used for specific applications.

    - Weldments make ultrasonic testing difficult.

    - Lack of penetration will appear on the scope as a definite break or discontinuity resembling a crack and will give a very sharp reflection.

  - Eddy Current Testing Method

    - Normally used to determine lack of penetration in nonferrous welded pipe and tubing.

- Eddy current testing can be used where other nonferrous articles can meet the configuration requirement of the equipment.

  – Magnetic Particle Testing Method

- Normally used where back side of weld is visible.

- Lack of penetration appears as an irregular indication of varying width.

  – Liquid Penetrant Testing Method

- Normally used where backside of weld is visible.

- Lack of penetration appears as an irregular indication of varying width.

- Residue left by the penetrant and the developer could contaminate any rewelding operation.

Laminations

- Category - Inherent

- Material - Ferrous and Nonferrous Wrought Material

- Discontinuity Characteristics

Surface and internal. Flat, extremely thin, generally aligned parallel to the work surface of the material. May contain a thin film of oxide between the surfaces. Found in forged, extruded and rolled material (Figure A-21).

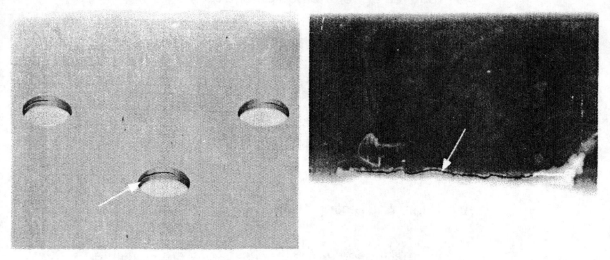

A   LAMINATION IN 0.250 IN. PLATE

B   LAMINATION IN 0.040 TITANIUM SHEET

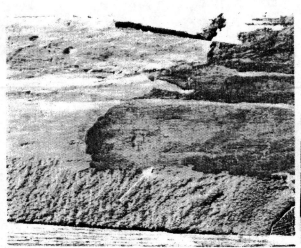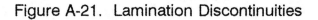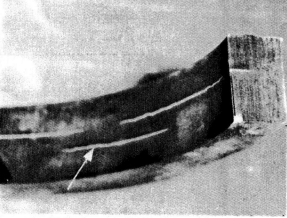

C   LAMINATION IN PLATE SHOWING SURFACE
ORIENTATION

D   LAMINATION IN 1 IN. BAR SHOWING SURFACE
ORIENTATION

Figure A-21. Lamination Discontinuities

- Metallurgical Analysis

  Laminations are separations or weaknesses generally aligned parallel to the work surface of the material. They may be the result of pipe, blister, seam, inclusions, or segregations elongated and made directional by working. Laminations are flattened impurities that are extremely thin.

- NDT Methods Application and Limitations

  - Ultrasonic Testing Method

    - For heavier gauge material, the geometry and orientation of lamination (normal to the beam) makes their detection limited to ultrasonic testing.

    - Numerous wave modes may be used, depending upon the material thickness or method selected for testing. Automatic and manual contact or immersion methods are adaptable.

    - Laminations appear as a definite interface with a loss of back reflection.

    - Through-transmission and reflection techniques are applicable for very thin sections.

  - Magnetic Particle Testing Method

    - Articles fabricated from ferromagnetic materials are normally tested for lamination by magnetic particle testing methods.

- Magnetic indication will appear as a straight, intermittent indication.

- Magnetic particle testing is not capable of determining the overall size or depth of the lamination.

- Liquid Penetrant Testing Method

  - Normally used on nonferrous materials.

  - Machining, honing, lapping, or blasting may smear the surface of the material and thereby close or mask surface lamination.

  - Acid and alkalines seriously limit the effectiveness of liquid penetrant testing. Thorough cleaning of the surface is essential.

- Eddy Current Testing Method

  - Not normally used to detect laminations.

- Radiographic Testing Method

  - Not recommended for detecting laminations. Laminations have very small thickness changes in the direction of the X-ray beam thereby making radiographic detection almost impossible.

Laps and Seams

- Category - Processing

- Material - Ferrous and Nonferrous Rolled Threads

- Discontinuity Characteristics

  Surface. Wavy lines, often quite deep and sometimes very tight, appearing as hairline cracks. Found in rolled threads in the minor pitch and major diameter of the thread and in direction of rolling (Figure A-22).

- Metallurgical Analysis

  During the rolling operation, faulty or oversized dies or an overfill of material may cause material to be folded over and flattened into the surface of the thread but not fused.

- NDT Methods Application and Limitations

  - Liquid Penetrant Testing Method

    - Compatibility with both ferrous and nonferrous materials makes fluorescent liquid penetrant the first choice.

    - Liquid penetrant indications will be circumferential, slightly curved, intermittent, or continuous indications. Laps and seams may occur individually or in clusters.

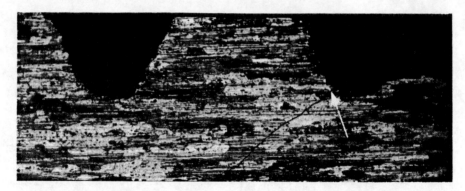

A TYPICAL AREAS OF FAILURE LAPS AND SEAMS

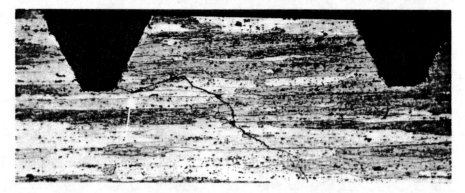

B FAILURE OCCURRING AT ROOT OF THREAD

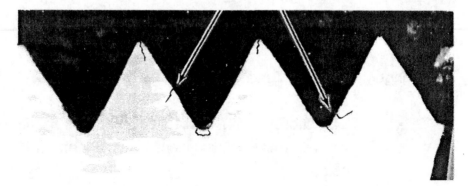

C AREAS WHERE LAPS AND SEAMS USUALLY OCCUR

Figure A-22. Lap and Seam Discontinuities in Rolled Threads

- Foreign material may not only interfere with the penetration of the penetrant into the discontinuity, but may cause an accumulation of penetrant in a nondefective area.

- Surface of threads may be smeared due to rolling operation, thereby sealing off laps and seams.

- Fluorescent and dye penetrants are not compatible. Dye penetrants tend to kill the fluorescent qualities in fluorescent penetrants.

– Magnetic Particle Testing Method

- Magnetic particle indications of laps and seams generally appear the same as liquid penetrant indications.

- Nonrelevant magnetic indications may result from threads.

- Questionable magnetic particle indications can be verified by liquid penetrant testing.

– Eddy Current Testing Method

- Probe coil design must match sample geometry.

– Ultrasonic Testing Method

- Not recommended for detecting laps and seams. Thread configurations restrict ultrasonic capability.

- Radiographic Testing Method

  - Not recommended for detecting laps and seams. Size and orientation of discontinuities restrict the capability of radiographic testing.

Laps and Seams

- Category - Processing

- Material - Ferrous and Nonferrous Wrought Material

- Discontinuity Characteristics

  - Lap Surface. Wavy lines which are usually not very pronounced nor tightly adherent since they usually enter the surface at a small angle. Laps may have surface openings which are smeared closed. Found in wrought forgings, plate, tubing, bar, and rod (Figure A-23).

  - Seam Surface. Lengthy, often quite deep, and sometimes very tight. Usually occur in fissures parallel with the grain, and, when associated with rolled rod and tubing, they may at times be spiral.

- Metallurgical Analysis

  Seams originate from blowholes, cracks, splits, and tears introduced in earlier processing and elongated in the direction of rolling or forging. The distance between adjacent interfaces of the discontinuity is very small.

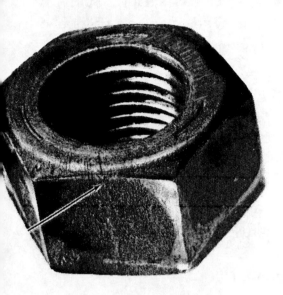
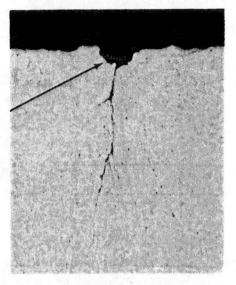

A   TYPICAL FORGING LAP   B   MICROGRAPH OF A LAP

Figure A-23. Lap and Seam Discontinuities in Wrought Material

Laps are similar to seams and may result from improper rolling,
forging, or sizing operations. Corners may be folded over during
the processing of the material or an overfill may exist during sizing
that results in the material being flattened but not fused into the
surface. Laps may occur on any part of the article.

• NDT Methods Application and Limitations

    — Magnetic Particle Testing Method

        • Magnetic particle testing is recommended for
          ferromagnetic material.

        • Surface and near-surface laps and seams may be
          detected by this method.

- Laps and seams may appear as straight, spiral, or slightly curved indications. They may be individual or clustered and continuous or intermittent.

- Magnetic buildup at laps and seams is very small; therefore, a magnetizing current greater than that used for the detection of cracks is necessary.

- Correct magnetizing technique should be used when examining for forging laps since the discontinuity may lie in a plane nearly parallel to the surface.

- Liquid Penetrant Testing Method

  - Liquid penetrant testing is recommended for nonferrous material.

  - Laps and seams may be very tight and difficult to detect, especially by liquid penetrant.

  - Liquid penetrant testing of laps and seams can be improved slightly by heating the article before applying the penetrant.

- Ultrasonic Testing Method

  - Normally used to test wrought material prior to machining.

  - Surface wave and/or time-of-flight techniques permit accurate evaluation of the depth, length, and size of laps and seams.

- Ultrasonic indications of laps and seams will appear as definite interfaces within the metal.

- Eddy Current Testing Method

  - Normally used for the evaluation of laps and seams in tubing and pipe.

  - Other articles can be screened by eddy current where article configuration and size permit.

- Radiographic Testing Method

  - Not recommended for detecting laps and seams in wrought material.

Microshrinkage

- Category - Processing

- Material - Magnesium Casting

- Discontinuity Characteristics

  Internal. Small filamentary voids in the grain boundaries appear as concentrated porosity in cross section (Figure A-24).

- Metallurgical Analysis

  Shrinkage occurs while the metal is in a plastic or semimolten state. If sufficient molten metal cannot flow into different areas as it cools, the shrinkage will leave a void. The void is identified by its appearance and by the time it occurs in the plastic range. Microshrinkage is caused by the withdrawal of the low melting point constituent from the grain boundaries.

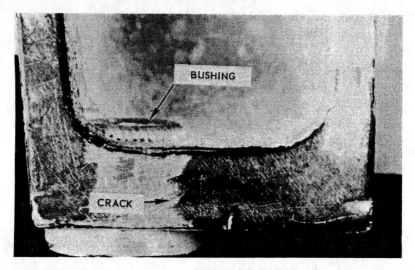

A   CRACKED MAGNESIUM HOUSING

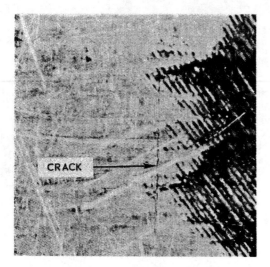

B   CLOSE-UP VIEW OF (A)

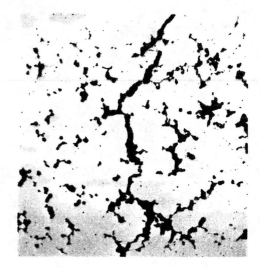

C   MICROGRAPH OF CRACKED AREA

Figure A-24.   Microshrinkage Discontinuity

- NDT Methods Application and Limitations

    - Radiographic Testing Method

        • Radiography is universally used to determine the acceptance level of microshrinkage.

        • Microshrinkage will appear on the radiograph as an elongated swirl resembling feathery streaks or as dark, irregular patches that are indicative of cavities in the grain boundaries.

    - Liquid Penetrant Testing Method

        • Normally used on finished machined surfaces.

        • Microshrinkage is not normally open to the surface; therefore, these conditions will be detected in machined areas.

        • The appearance of the indication depends on the plane through which the microshrinkage has been cut. The appearance varies from a continuous hairline to a massive porous indication.

        • Penetrant may act as a contaminant by saturating the microporous casting, affecting its ability to accept a surface treatment.

        • Serious structural or dimensional damage to the article can result from the improper use of acids or alkalies. They should never be used unless approval is obtained.

- Eddy Current Testing Method

    • Not recommended for detecting microshrinkage. Article configuration and type of discontinuity do not lend themselves to eddy current testing.

- Ultrasonic Testing Method

    • Not recommended for detecting microshrinkage. Cast structure and article configuration are restricting factors.

- Magnetic Particle Testing Method

    • Not applicable. Material is nonferrous.

Gas Porosity

• Category - Processing

• Material - Ferrous and Nonferrous Weldments

• Discontinuity Characteristics

Surface or subsurface. Rounded or elongated, teardrop-shaped, with or without a sharp discontinuity at the point. Scattered uniformly throughout the weld or isolated in small groups. May also be concentrated at the root or toe (Figure A-25).

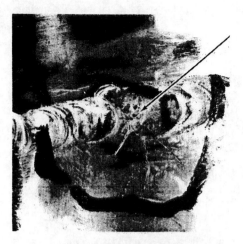

A TYPICAL SURFACE POROSITY

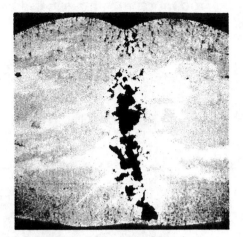

B CROSS SECTION OF (A) SHOWING EXTENT OF POROSITY

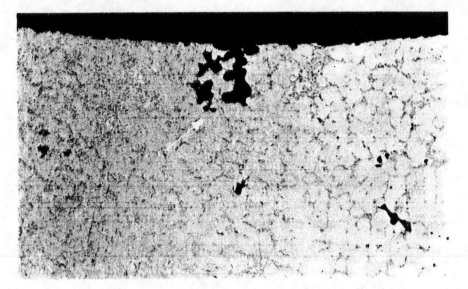

C MICROGRAPH OF CROSS SECTION SHOWING TYPICAL SHRINKAGE POROSITY

Figure A-25. Gas Porosity Discontinuity

● Metallurgical Analysis

Porosity in welds is caused by gas entrapment in the molten metal, too much moisture on the base or filler metal, or improper cleaning or preheating.

- NDT Methods Application and Limitations

    - Radiography Testing Method

        - Radiography is the most universally used NDT method for the detection of gas porosity in weldments.

        - The radiographic image of a "round" porosity will appear as oval-shaped spots with smooth edges, while "elongated" porosity will appear as oval-shaped spots with the major axis sometimes several times longer than the minor axis.

        - Foreign material such as loose scale, flux, or splatter will affect validity of test results.

    - Ultrasonic Testing Method

        - Ultrasonic testing equipment is highly sensitive and is capable of detecting microseparations. Established standards should be used if valid test results are to be obtained.

        - Surface finish and grain size will affect the validity of the test results.

- Eddy Current Testing Method

    • Normally confined to thin-walled welded pipe and tube.

    • Penetration restricts testing to a depth of more than 0.25 inch (6.35 mm).

- Liquid Penetrant Testing Method

    • Normally confined to in-process control of ferrous and nonferrous weldments.

    • Liquid penetrant testing, like magnetic particle testing, is restricted to surface evaluation.

    • Extreme caution must be exercised to prevent any cleaning material, magnetic (iron oxide), and liquid penetrant materials from becoming entrapped and contaminating the rewelding operation.

- Magnetic Particle Testing Method

    • Not normally used to detect gas porosity. Only surface porosity would be evident. Near surface porosity would not be clearly defined since indications are neither strong nor pronounced.

Unfused Porosity

• Category - Processing

- Material - Aluminum

- Discontinuity Characteristics

  Internal. Wafer-thin fissures aligned parallel with the grain flow. Found in wrought aluminum that has been rolled, forged or extruded (Figure A-26).

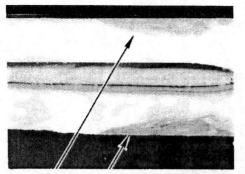
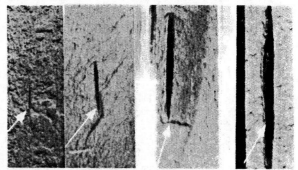

A. FRACTURED SPECIMEN SHOWING UNFUSED POROSITY

B. UNFUSED POROSITY EQUIVALENT TO 1/64 IN. (0.40 mm), 3/64 IN. (1.17 mm) 5/64 IN. (1.98 mm) AND 8/64 IN. (3.18 mm) (left to right)

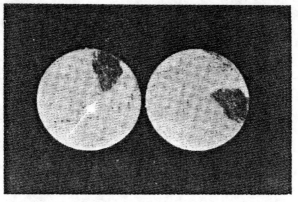

C. TYPICAL UNFUSED POROSITY

Figure A-26. Unfused Porosity Discontinuity

- Metallurgical Analysis

  Unfused porosity is attributed to porosity in the cast ingot. During the rolling, forging or extruding operations it is flattened into a wafer-

A-72

thin shape. If the internal surface of these discontinuities is oxidized or is composed of a foreign material, they will not fuse during the subsequent processing. This results in an extremely thin interface or void.

- NDT Methods Application and Limitations

  - Ultrasonic Testing Method

    - Used extensively for the detection of unfused porosity.

    - Raw materials may be tested in the "as-received" configuration.

    - Ultrasonic testing fixes the location of the void in all three directions.

    - Where the general direction of the discontinuity is unknown, it may be necessary to test from several directions.

    - Method of manufacture and subsequent article configuration will determine the orientation of the unfused porosity to the material surface.

  - Liquid Penetrant Testing Method

    - Normally used on nonferrous machined articles.

    - Unfused porosity will appear as a straight line of varying lengths running parallel with the grain. Liquid penetrant testing is restricted to surface evaluation.

- Surface preparations such as vapor blasting, honing, grinding, or sanding may obliterate possible indications by masking the surface discontinuities and thereby restricting the reliability of liquid penetrant testing.

- Excessive agitation of penetrant materials may produce foaming.

    – Eddy Current Testing Method

- Not normally used for detecting unfused porosity.

    – Radiographic Testing Method

- Not normally used for detecting unfused porosity. Wafer-thin discontinuities are difficult to detect by a method that measures density or that requires that the discontinuity be perpendicular to the X-ray beam.

    – Magnetic Particle Testing Method

- Not applicable. Material is nonferrous.

Stress Corrosion

- Category - Service

- Material - Ferrous and Nonferrous

- Discontinuity Characteristics

— Surface. Range from shallow to very deep, and usually follow the grain flow of the material; however, transverse cracks are also possible (Figure A-27).

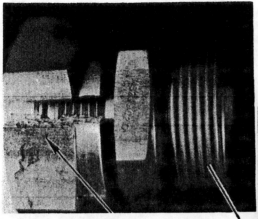
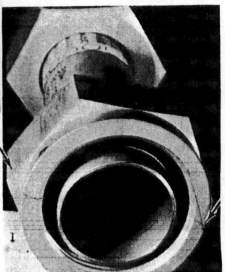

FRACTURED ALUMINUM ALLOY COUPLING
DUE TO STRESS CORROSION

Figure A-27. Stress Corrosion Discontinuity

• Metallurgical Analysis

The following three factors are necessary for the phenomenon of stress corrosion to occur: 1) a sustained static tensile stress, 2) the presence of a corrosive environment, and 3) the use of a material that is susceptible to this type of failure. Stress corrosion is much more likely to occur at high levels of stress than at low levels of stress. The type of stresses include residual (internal) as well as those from external (applied) loading.

- NDT Methods Application and Limitations

  - Liquid Penetrant Testing Method

    - Liquid penetrant is normally used for the detection of stress corrosion.

    - In the preparation, application, and final cleaning of articles, extreme care must be exercised to prevent overspraying and contamination of the surrounding articles.

    - Chemical cleaning immediately before the application of liquid penetrant may seriously affect the test results if the solvents are not given time to evaporate.

    - Service articles may contain moisture within the discontinuity which will dilute, contaminate, and invalidate results if the moisture is not removed.

  - Ultrasonic Testing Method

    - Advanced techniques have been successfully used to detect stress corrosion and stress corrosion cracking in the nuclear industry.

    - Indications appear in a variety of amplitudes, shapes, and characteristics.

    - Interpretation is often difficult, requiring highly-trained operators.

- Eddy Current Testing Method

    • Eddy current equipment is capable of resolving stress corrosion where article configuration is compatible with equipment limitations.

- Magnetic Particle Testing Method

    • Not normally used to detect stress corrosion. Configuration of article and usual nonferromagnetic condition exclude magnetic particle testing.

- Radiographic Testing Method

    • Not normally used to detect stress corrosion. Surface indications are best detected by NDT method designed for such applications; however, radiography can and has shown stress corrosion with the use of the proper technique.

Hydraulic Tubing

- Category - Processing and Service

- Material - Aluminum

- Discontinuity Characteristics

Surface and internal. Range in size from short to long, shallow to very tight and deep. Usually they will be found in the direction of the grain flow with the exception of stress corrosion which has no direction (Figure A-28).

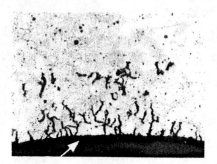

A   INTERGRANULAR CORROSION

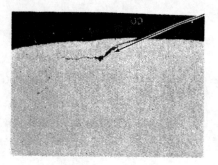

B   LAP IN OUTER SURFACE OF TUBING

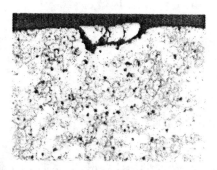

C   EMBEDDED FOREIGN MATERIAL

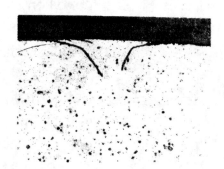

D   TWIN LAPS IN OUTER SURFACE OF TUBING

Figure A-28.   Hydraulic Tubing Discontinuities

●   Metallurgical Analysis

Hydraulic tubing discontinuities are usually one of the following.

−   Foreign material coming in contact with the tube material and being embedded into the surface of the tube.

−   Laps which are the result of material being folded over and not fused.

- Seams which originate from blowholes, cracks, splits, and tears introduced in the earlier processing, and then are elongated during rolling.

- Intergranular corrosion which is due to the presence of a corrosive environment.

- NDT Methods Application and Limitations

    - Eddy Current Testing Method

        • Universally used for testing of nonferrous tubing.

        • Heavier-walled tubing (0.25 inch or 6.35 mm and over) may not be successfully tested due to the penetration ability of the equipment.

        • The specific nature of various discontinuities may not be clearly defined.

        • Test results will not be valid unless controlled by known standards.

        • Testing of ferromagnetic material may be difficult.

        • All material should be free of any foreign material that would invalidate the test results.

    - Liquid Penetrant Testing Method

        • Not normally used for detecting tubing discontinuities. Eddy current is more economical, faster, and, with established standards, is more reliable.

- Ultrasonic Testing Method

    • Not normally used for detecting tubing discontinuities. Eddy current is recommended over ultrasonic testing since it is faster and more economical for this range of surface discontinuity and nonferrous material.

- Radiographic Testing Method

    • Not normally used for detecting tubing discontinuities. The size and type of discontinuity and the configuration of the article limit the use of radiography for screening of material for this group of discontinuities.

- Magnetic Particle Testing Method

    • Not applicable. Material is nonferrous.

Mandrel Drag

- Category - Processing

- Material - Nonferrous, Thick-walled Seamless Tubing

- Discontinuity Characteristics

Internal surface of thick-walled tubing. Range from shallow, even gouges to ragged tears. Often a slug of the material will be embedded within the gouged area (Figure A-29).

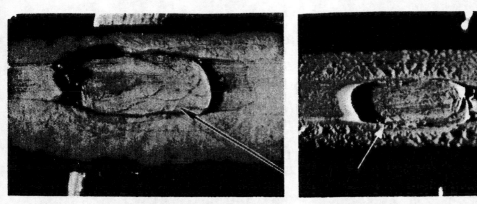

A. EMBEDDED SLUG SHOWING DEEP GOUGE MARKS   B. SLUG BROKEN LOOSE FROM TUBING WALL

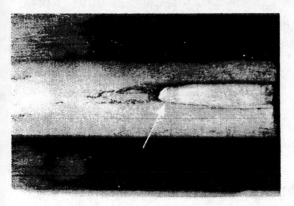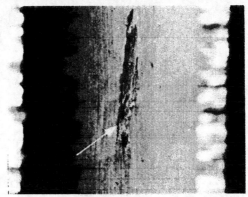

C. ANOTHER TYPE OF EMBEDDED SLUG   D. GOUGE ON INNER SURFACE OF PIPE

Figure A-29. Mandrel Drag Discontinuities

● Metallurgical Analysis

During the manufacture of thick-walled seamless tubing, the billet is ruptured as it passes through the offset rolls. As the piercing mandrel follows this fracture, a portion of the material may break loose and be forced over the mandrel. As it does, the surface of the tubing may be scored or have the slug embedded into the wall. Certain types of material are more prone to this type of failure than others.

- NDT Methods Application and Limitations

  - Eddy Current Testing Method

    - Normally used for the testing of thin-walled pipe or tube.

    - Eddy current testing may be confined to nonferrous materials.

    - Discontinuities are qualitative indications and not quantitative indications.

    - Several factors simultaneously affect output indications.

  - Ultrasonic Testing Method

    - Normally used for the screening of thick-walled pipe or tube for mandrel drag.

    - Can be used to test both ferrous and nonferrous pipe or tube.

    - May be used in support of production line, since it is adaptable for automatic instrumentation.

    - Configuration of mandrel drag or tear will produce very sharp and noticeable indications on the scope.

  - Radiographic Testing Method

    - Not normally used although it has been instrumental

in the detection of mandrel drag during examination of adjacent welds. Complete coverage requires several exposures around the circumference of the tube. This method is not designed for production support since it is very slow and costly for large volumes of pipe or tube. Radiograph will disclose only two dimensions and not the third.

— Liquid Penetrant Testing Method

• Not recommended for detecting mandrel drag since discontinuity is internal and would not be detectable.

— Magnetic Particle Testing Method

• Not recommended for detecting mandrel drag. Discontinuities are not close enough to the surface to be detectable by magnetic particles. Most mandrel drag will occur in seamless stainless steel.

Semiconductors

• Category - Processing and Service

• Material - Hardware

• Discontinuity Characteristics

Internal. Appear in many sizes and shapes and various degrees of density. They may be misformed, misaligned, damaged, or may have broken internal hardware. Found in transistors, diodes, resistors, and capacitors (Figure A-30).

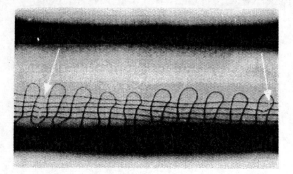

A. STRANDS BROKEN IN HEATER BLANKET

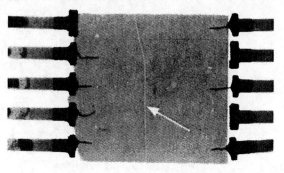

B. FINE CRACK IN PLASTIC CASING MATERIAL

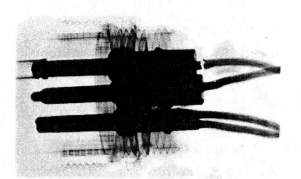

C. BROKEN ELECTRICAL CABLE

D. FOREIGN MATERIAL WITHIN SEMICONDUCTOR

Figure A-30. Semiconductor Discontinuities

- Metallurgical Analysis

  Semiconductor discontinuities such as loose wire, weld splash, flakes, solder balls, loose leads, inadequate clearance between internal elements and case and inclusions or voids in seals or around lead connections are the product of processing errors.

- NDT Methods Application and Limitations

  - Radiographic Testing Method

- Universally used as the NDT method for the detection of discontinuities in semiconductors.

- The configuration and internal structure of the various semiconductors limit the NDT method of radiography.

- Semiconductors that have copper heat sinks may require more than one technique due to the density of the copper.

- Internal wires in semiconductors are very fine and may be constructed from materials of different density such as copper, silver, gold, and aluminum. If the latter is used with the others, special techniques may be needed to resolve test reliability.

- Microparticles may require the highest sensitivity to resolve.

- The complexity of the internal structure of semiconductors may require additional views to exclude the possibility of nondetection of discontinuities due to masking by hardware.

- Positive positioning of each semiconductor will prevent invalid interpretation.

- Source angle should give minimum distortion.

- Preliminary examination of semiconductors may be accomplished using a vidicon system that would allow visual observation during 360° rotation of the article.

- Eddy Current Testing Method

    • Not recommended for detecting semiconductor discontinuities. Nature of discontinuity and method of construction of the article do not lend themselves to this form of NDT.

- Magnetic Particle Testing Method

    • Not recommended for detecting semiconductor discontinuities.

- Liquid Penetrant Testing Method

    • Not recommended for detecting semiconductor discontinuities.

- Ultrasonic Testing Method

    • Not recommended for detecting semiconductor discontinuities.

Hot Tears

• Category - Inherent

• Material - Ferrous Castings

• Discontinuity Characteristics

Internal or near surface. Appear as ragged line of variable width and numerous branches. Occur individually or in groups (Figure A-31).

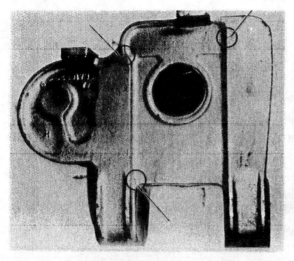

A. TYPICAL HOT TEARS IN CASTING

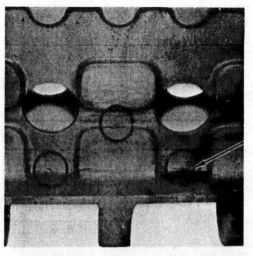

B. HOT TEARS IN FILLET OF CASTING

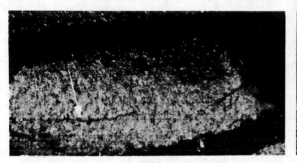

C. CLOSE-UP OF HOT TEARS IN (A)

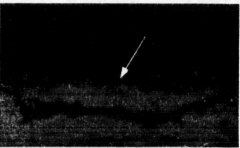

D. CLOSE-UP OF HOT TEARS IN (B)

Figure A-31. Hot Tear Discontinuities

- Metallurgical Analysis

Hot cracks (tears) are caused by nonuniform cooling resulting in stresses which rupture the surface of the metal while its temperature is still in the brittle range. Tears may originate where stresses are set up by the more rapid cooling of thin sections that adjoin heavier masses of metal which are slower to cool.

- NDT Methods Application and Limitations

  - Radiographic Testing Method

    - Radiographic testing is the first choice since the material is cast structure and the discontinuities may be internal and surface.

    - Orientation of the hot tear in relation to the source may influence the test results.

    - The sensitivity level may not be sufficient to detect fine surface hot tears.

  - Magnetic Particle Testing Method

    - Hot tears that are exposed to the surface can be screened with magnetic particle method.

    - Article configuration and metallurgical composition may make demagnetization difficult.

    - Although magnetic particle testing can detect near surface hot tears, radiography should be used for final analysis.

    - Foreign material not removed prior to testing will cause an invalid test.

- Liquid Penetrant Testing Method

    • Liquid penetrant testing is recommended for nonferrous cast material.

    • Method is confined to surface evaluation.

    • The use of penetrants on castings may act as a contaminant by saturating the porous structure and thereby affecting the ability to apply surface finish.

    • Repeatability of indications may be poor.

- Ultrasonic Testing Method

    • Not recommended for detecting hot tears. Discontinuities of this type, when associated with cast structure, do not lend themselves to ultrasonic testing.

- Eddy Current Testing Method

    • Capable of detecting surface hot tears. Metallurgical structure, along with the complex configurations, may require specialized probes and techniques.

Intergranular Corrosion

• Category - Service

• Material - Nonferrous

- Discontinuity Characteristics

  Surface or internal. A series of small micro-openings with no definite pattern. May appear individually or in groups. The insidious nature of intergranular corrosion results from the fact that very little corrosion or corrosion product is visible on the surface. Intergranular corrosion may extend in any direction following the grain boundaries of the material (Figure A-32).

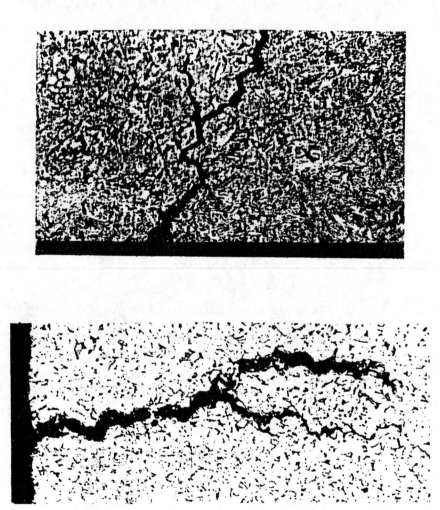

Figure A-32. Intergranular Corrosion Discontinuities

- Metallurgical Analysis

  Two factors that contribute to intergranular corrosion are:

  - Metallurgical structure of the material that is prone to intergranular corrosion, such as unstabilized 300 series stainless steel.

  - Improper stress relieving or heat treat may create the susceptibility to intergranular corrosion.

  Either of these conditions, coupled with a corrosive atmosphere, will result in intergranular attack.

- NDT Methods Application and Limitations

  - Liquid Penetrant Testing Method

    - Liquid Penetrant testing is the first choice due to the size and location of this type of discontinuity.

    - Chemical cleaning operations immediately before the application of liquid penetrant may contaminate the article and seriously affect test results.

    - Cleaning with solvents may release chlorine and accelerate intergranular corrosion.

    - Trapped penetrant solution may present a cleaning or removal problem.

–　　Ultrasonic Testing Method

- Advanced techniques have been successfully used to detect stress corrosion and stress corrosion cracking in the nuclear industry.

- Indications appear in a variety of amplitudes, shapes, and characteristics lending difficult interpretation.

–　　Eddy Current Testing Method

- Eddy current can be used for the screening of intergranular corrosion.

- Tube or pipe lend themselves readily to this method of NDT testing.

- Metallurgical structure of the material may seriously affect the output indications.

–　　Radiographic Testing Method

- Intergranular corrosion in the more advanced stages has been detected with radiography.

- Sensitivity levels may prevent the detection of fine intergranular corrosion.

- Radiography may not indicate the surface on which the intergranular corrosion occurs.

– Magnetic Particle Testing Method

- Not recommended for detecting intergranular corrosion. Type of discontinuity and material restrict the use of magnetic particles.

APPENDIX B

GLOSSARY

A-scan Display   A display in which the received signal is displayed as a vertical displacement from the horizontal sweep time trace, while the horizontal distance between any two signals represents the sound-path distance (or time of travel) between the two.

Absorption Coefficient, Linear   The fractional decrease in transmitted intensity per unit of absorber thickness. It is usually designated by the symbol μ and expressed in units of cm^{-1}.

Acceptance Standard   A control specimen containing natural or artificial discontinuities that are well defined and, in size or extent, similar to the maximum acceptable in the product. Also may refer to the document defining acceptable discontinuity size limits.

Acoustic Impedance   The factor which controls the propagation of an ultrasonic wave at a boundary interface. It is the product of the material density and the acoustic wave velocity within that material.

Amplifier   A device to increase or amplify electrical impulses.

Amplitude, Indication   The vertical height of a received indication, measured from base-to-peak or peak-to-peak.

Angle Beam Testing   A testing method in which transmission is at an angle to the sound entry surface.

Angle of Incidence   The angle between the incident (transmitted) beam and a normal to the boundary interface.

Angle of Reflection   The angle between the reflected beam and a normal to the boundary interface. The angle of reflection is equal to the angle of incidence.

Angle of Refraction   The angle between the refracted rays of an ultrasonic beam and the normal (or perpendicular line) to the refracting surface.

Angle Transducer   A transducer that transmits or receives the acoustic energy at an acute angle to the surface to achieve a specific effect such as the setting up of shear or surface waves in the part being inspected.

Anisotropic   A condition in which properties of a medium (velocity, for example) vary according to the direction in which they are measured.

Array Transducer   A transducer made up of several piezoelectric elements individually connected so that the signals they transmit or receive may be treated separately or combined as desired.

ANSI   American National Standards Institute

API   American Petroleum Institute

ASME   American Society of Mechanical Engineers

ASNT   American Society for Nondestructive Testing

ASTM   American Society for Testing and Materials

Attenuation Coefficient   A factor which is determined by the degree of scatter or absorption of ultrasound energy per unit distance traveled.

Attenuation   The loss in acoustic energy which occurs between any two points of travel. This loss may be due to absorption, reflection, scattering, etc.

Attenuator   A device for measuring attenuation, usually calibrated in decibels (dB).

B-scan Display   A data presentation method that represents a cross-sectional or end view display of the test article.

Back Reflection   The signal received from the back surface of a test object. Also referred to as back wall reflection.

Back Scatter   Scattered signals that are directed back to the transmitter/receiver.

Background Noise   Extraneous signals caused by signal sources within the ultrasonic testing system, including the material in test.

Baseline   The horizontal line across the bottom of the CRT created by the sweep circuit.

Basic Calibration   The procedure of standardizing an instrument using calibration reflectors described in an application document.

Beam Exit/Index Point   The point on a transducer (primarily angle beam) indicating the physical location through which the emergent beam axis passes.

Beam Spread   The divergence of the sound beam as it travels through a medium.

Bi-modal   The propagation of sound in a test article where at least a shear wave and a longitudinal wave exists. The operation of angle beam testing at less than first critical angle.

Boundary Indication A reflection of an ultrasonic beam from an interface.

Broad Banded   Having a relatively wide frequency bandwidth. Used to describe pulses which display a wide frequency spectrum and receivers capable of amplifying them.

C-scan A data presentation method yielding a plan (top) view through the scanned surface of the part. Through gating, only indications arising from the interior of the test object are indicated.

Calibration   To determine or mark the graduations of the ultrasonic system's display relative to a known standard or reference.

Calibration Reflector   A reflector with a known dimensioned surface established to provide an accurately reproducible reference.

Collimator   An attachment designed to reduce the ultrasonic beam spread.

Compensator   An electrical matching network to compensate for circuit impedance differences.

Compressional Wave   A wave in which the particle motion or vibration is in the same direction as the propagated wave (longitudinal wave).

Contact Testing   A technique of testing in which the transducer contacts the test surface, either directly or through a thin layer of couplant.

Contact Transducer   A transducer which is coupled to a test surface either directly or through a thin film of couplant.

Continuous Wave   A wave that continues without interruption.

Contracted Sweep   A contraction of the horizontal sweep on the viewing screen of the ultrasonic instrument.   Contraction of this sweep permits viewing reflections occurring over a greater sound-path distance or duration of time.

Corner Effect   The strong reflection obtained when an ultrasonic beam is directed toward the inner section of two or three mutually perpendicular surfaces.

Couplant   A substance used between the face of the transducer and test surface to permit or improve transmission of ultrasonic energy across this boundary or interface.   Primarily used to remove the air in the interface.

Critical Angle   The incident angle of the sound beam beyond which a specific refracted mode of vibration no longer exists.

Cross Talk   An unwanted condition in which acoustic energy is coupled from the transmitting crystal to the receiving crystal without propagating along the intended path through the material.

Damping (transducer)   Limiting the duration of vibration in the search unit by either electrical or mechanical means.

Dead Zone   The distance in a material from the sound entry surface to the nearest inspectable sound path.

Decibel (dB)   The logarithmic expression of a ratio of two amplitudes or intensities of acoustic energy.

Defect/Flaw   A material discontinuity whose size, shape, orientation, or location make it detrimental to the useful service of the test object or component.

Defect Indication   The oscilloscope presentation of the energy returned by a rejectable flaw in the material.

Delamination   A laminar discontinuity, generally an area of unbonded materials.

Delay Line   A material (liquid or solid) placed in front of a transducer to cause a time delay between the initial pulse and the front surface reflection.

Delayed Sweep   A means of delaying the start of horizontal sweep, thereby eliminating the presentation of early response data.

Delta Effect   Acoustic energy re-radiated by a discontinuity.

Detectability   The ability of the ultrasonic system to locate a discontinuity.

Diffraction   The deflection, or "bending," of a wave front when passing the edge or edges of a discontinuity.

Diffuse Reflection   Scattered, incoherent reflections caused by rough surfaces or associate interface reflection of ultrasonic waves from irregularities of the same order of magnitude or greater than the wavelength.

Discontinuity   An interruption or change in the physical structure or characteristics of a material.

Dispersion, Sound   Scattering of an ultrasonic beam as a result of diffused reflection from a highly-irregular surface.

Distance Amplitude Correction (DAC)   Compensation of gain as a function of time for difference in amplitude of reflections from equal reflectors at different sound travel distances.   Also referred to as time corrected gain (TCG), time variable gain (TVG) and sensitivity time control (STC).

Divergence   Spreading of ultrasonic waves after leaving search unit, and is a function of diameter and frequency.

Dual-Element Technique   The technique of ultrasonic testing using two transducers with one acting as the transmitter and one as the receiver.

Dual-Element Transducer   A single transducer housing containing two piezoelectric elements, one for transmitting and one for receiving.

Echo   See **Boundary Indication**.

Effective Penetration   The maximum depth in a material at which the ultrasonic transmission is sufficient for proper detection of discontinuities.

Electrical Noise   Extraneous signals caused by externally radiated electrical signals or from electrical interferences within the ultrasonic instrumentation.

Electromagnetic Acoustic Transducer (EMAT)   A device using the magneto effect to generate and receive acoustic signals for ultrasonic nondestructive tests.

Evaluation   The process of deciding the severity of a condition after an indication has been interpreted.   Evaluation determines if the test object should be rejected, repaired, accepted, or replaced.

Far Field   The region beyond the near field in which areas of high and low acoustic intensity cease to occur.

First Leg   The sound path beginning at the exit point of the probe and extending to the point of contact opposite the examination surface when performing angle beam testing.

Focused Transducer   A transducer with a concave face which converges the acoustic beam to a focal point or line at a defined distance from the face.

Focusing   Concentration or convergence of energy into a smaller beam.

Fraunhofer Zone   See **Far Field**.

Frequency   Number of complete cycles of a wave motion passing a given point in a unit time (1 second); number of times a vibration is repeated at the same point in the same direction per unit time (usually per second).

Fresnel Field   See **Near Field**.

Gate   An electronic means to monitor an associated segment of time, distance, or impulse.

Ghost   An indication which has no direct relation to reflected pulses from discontinuities in the materials being tested.

Hertz (Hz)   One cycle per second.

Horizontal Sweep   See **Baseline**.

Horizontal Linearity   A measure of the proportionality between the positions of the indications appearing on the baseline and the positions of their sources.

Immersion Testing   A technique of testing, using a liquid as an ultrasonic couplant, in which the test part and at least the transducer face is immersed in the couplant and the transducer is not in contact with the test part.

Impedance (acoustic)   A material characteristic defined as a product of particle velocity and material density.

Indication (ultrasonics)   The signal displayed or read on the ultrasonic systems display.

Initial Pulse   The first indication which may appear on the screen. This indication represents the emission of ultrasonic energy from the crystal face (main bang).

Interface   The physical boundary between two adjacent acoustic mediums.

Insonification   Irradiation with sound.

Interpretation   The determination of the source and relevancy of an indication.

Isotropy   A condition in which significant medium properties (velocity, for example) are the same in all directions.

Lamb Wave   A type of ultrasonic vibration guided by parallel surfaces of thin mediums capable of propagation in different modes.

Linearity (area)   A system response in which a linear relationship exists between amplitude of response and the discontinuity sizes being evaluated (necessarily limited by the size of the ultrasonic beam).

Linearity (depth)   A system response where a linear relationship exists with varying depth for a constant size discontinuity.

Longitudinal Wave   See **Compressional Wave**.

Longitudinal Wave Velocity   The unit speed of propagation of a longitudinal (compressional) wave through a material.

Loss of Back Reflection   Absence of or a significant reduction of an indication from the back surface of the article being inspected.

Major Screen Divisions   The vertical graticule used to divide the CRT into 10 equal horizontal segments.

Manipulator   A device used to orient the transducer assembly.   As applied to immersion techniques, it provides either angular or normal incidence and fixes the transducer-to-part distance.

Material Noise   Extraneous signals caused by the structure of the material being tested.

Miniature Angle Beam Block   A specific type of reference standard used primarily for the angle beam method, but also used for straight beam and surface wave tests.

Minor Screen Divisions   The vertical graticule used to divide the CRT into 50 equal segments.   Each major screen division is divided into 5 equal segments or minor divisions.

Mode Conversion The change of ultrasonic wave propagation upon reflection or refraction at acute angles at an interface.

Mode The manner in which acoustic energy is propagated through a material as characterized by the particle motion of the wave.

Multiple Back Reflections Repetitive indications from the back surface of the material being examined.

Nanosecond One billionth (10^{-9}) of a second.

Narrow Banded A relative term denoting a restricted range of frequency response.

Near Field A distance immediately in front of a transducer composed of complex and changing wave front characteristics. Also known as the Fresnel field.

Node The point on the examination surface where the V-path begins or ends. (See **V-path**)

Noise Any undesired indications that tend to interfere with the interpretation or processing of the ultrasonic information; also referred to as "grass."

Nonrelevant Indication See **Ghost**.

Normal Incidence A condition where the angle of incidence is zero.

Orientation The angular relationship of a surface, plane, defect axis, etc., to a reference plane or sound entry surface.

Penetration (ultrasonic)   Propagation of ultrasonic energy through an article. See **Effective Penetration**.

Phased Array   A mosaic of probe elements in which the timing of the element's excitation can be individually controlled to produce certain desired effects, such as steering the beam axis or focusing the beam.

Piezoelectric Effect   The characteristic of certain materials to generate electrical charges when subjected to mechanical vibrations and, conversely, to generate mechanical vibrations when subjected to electrical pulses.

Pitch-Catch   See **Two-Probe Method**.

Polarized Ceramics   Ceramic materials that are sintered (pressed), heated (approximately 1000°C), and polarized by applying a direct voltage of a few thousand volts per centimeter of thickness. The polarization is the process that makes these ceramics piezoelectric.   Includes sodium bismuth titanate, lead metaniobate, and several materials based on lead zirconate titanate (PZT).

Presentation   The method used to show ultrasonic information. This may include (among others) A-, B-, or C-scans displayed on various types of recorders, CRTs, LCDs or computerized displays.

Probe   Transducer or search unit.

Propagation   Advancement of a wave through a medium.

Pulse-Echo Technique   An ultrasonic test technique using equipment which transmits a series of pulses separated by a constant period of time; i.e., energy is not sent out continuously.

Pulse Length   Time duration of the pulse from the search unit.

Pulse Rate   For the pulse-echo technique, the number of pulses transmitted in a unit of time (also called pulse repetition rate).

Radio Frequency Display (RF)   The presentation of unrectified signals in a display.

Range   The maximum ultrasonic path length that is displayed.

Rarefaction   The thinning out or moving apart of the consistent particles in the propagating medium due to the relaxation phase of an ultrasonic cycle.   Opposite in its effect to compression.   The sound wave is composed of alternate compressions and refractions of the particles in a material.

Rayleigh Wave/Surface Wave   A wave that travels on or close to the surface and readily follows the curvature of the part being examined. Reflections occur only at sharp changes of direction of the surface.

Receiver   The section of the ultrasonic instrument that amplifies the electronic signals returning from the test specimen.   Also, the probe that receives the reflected signals.

Reference Blocks   A block or series of blocks of material containing artificial or actual discontinuities of one or more reflecting areas at one or more distances from the sound entry surface.   These are used for calibrating instruments and in defining the size and distance of discontinuous areas in materials.

Reflection   The characteristic of a surface to change the direction of propagating acoustic energy; the return of sound waves from surfaces.

Refraction A change in the direction and velocity of acoustic energy after it has passed at an acute angle through an interface between two different mediums.

Refractive Index The ratio of the velocity of a incident wave to the velocity of the refracted wave. It is a measure of the amount a wave will be refracted when it enters the second medium after leaving the first.

Reject/Suppression An instrument function or control used for reducing low amplitude signals.   Use of this control may affect vertical linearity.

Relevant Indication In NDT, an indication from a discontinuity requiring evaluation.

Repetition Rate The rate at which the individual pulses of acoustic energy are generated; also **Pulse Rate**.

Resolving Power The capability measurement of an ultrasonic system to separate in time two closely-spaced discontinuities or to separate closely-spaced multiple reflections.

Resonance Technique A technique using the resonance principle for determining velocity, thickness or presence of laminar discontinuities.

Resonance The condition in which the frequency of a forcing vibration (ultrasonic wave) is the same as the natural vibration frequency of the propagation body (test object), resulting in large amplitude vibrations.

Saturation (scope) A term used to describe an indication of such a size as to exceed full screen height (100 percent).

Scanning (manual and automatic) The moving of the search unit or units along a test surface to obtain complete testing of a material.

Scattering   Dispersion of ultrasonic waves in a medium due to causes other than absorption. See **Diffuse** and **Dispersion**.

Second Leg   The sound path beginning at the point of contact on the opposite surface and extending to the point of contact on the examination surface when performing angle beam testing.

Sensitivity   The ability to detect small discontinuities at given distances. The level of amplification at which the receiving circuit in an ultrasonic instrument is set.

Shear Wave   The wave in which the particles of the medium vibrate in a direction perpendicular to the direction of propagation.

Signal-to-Noise Ratio (SNR)   The ratio of amplitudes of indications from the smallest discontinuity considered significant and those caused by random factors, such as heterogeneity in grain size, etc.

Skip Distance   In angle beam tests of plate, pipe, or welds, the linear or surface distance from the sound entry point to the first reflection point on the same surface.

Snell's Law   The law that defines the relationship between the angle of incidence and the angle of refraction across an interface, based on a change in ultrasonic velocity.

Specific Acoustic Impedance   A characteristic which acts to determine the amount of reflection which occurs at an interface and represents the wave velocity and the product of the density of the medium in which the wave is propagating.

Standardize   See **Calibration**.

Straight Beam An ultrasonic wave traveling normal to the test surface.

Surface Wave See **Rayleigh Wave**.

Sweep The uniform and repeated movement of a spot across the screen of a CRT to form the baseline.

Through-Transmission A test technique using two transducers in which the ultrasonic vibrations are emitted by one and received by the other, usually on the opposite side of the part. The ratio of the magnitudes of vibrations transmitted and received is used as the criterion of soundness.

Tip Diffraction The process by which a signal is generated from the tip (i.e., top of a fatigue crack) of a discontinuity through the interruption of an incident sound beam propagating through a material.

Transducer (search unit) An assembly consisting basically of a housing, piezoelectric element, backing material, wear plate (optional) and electrical leads for converting electrical impulses into mechanical energy and vice versa.

Transmission Angle The incident angle of the transmitted ultrasonic beam. It is zero degrees when the ultrasonic beam is perpendicular to the test surface.

Transmitter The electrical circuit of an ultrasonic instrument that generates the pulses emitted to the search unit. Also the probe that emits ultrasonic signals.

Transverse Wave See **Shear Wave**.

Two-Probe Method Use of two transducers for sending and receiving. May be either send-receive or through-transmission.

Ultrasonic Absorption   A damping of ultrasonic vibrations that occurs when the wave transverses a medium.

Ultrasonic Spectrum   The frequency span of elastic waves greater than the highest audible frequency, generally regarded as being higher than 20,000 hertz, to approximately 1000 megahertz.

Ultrasonic System   The totality of components utilized to perform an ultrasonic test on a test article.

Ultrasonic Testing   A nondestructive method of inspecting materials by the use of high-frequency sound waves into or through them.

V-path   The path of the ultrasonic beam in the test object from the point of entry on the examination surface to the back surface and reflecting to the front surface again.

Velocity   The speed at which sound travels through a medium.

Video Presentation   A CRT presentation in which radio frequency signals have been rectified and usually filtered.

Water Path   The distance from the face of the search unit to the entry surface of the material under test in immersion testing.

Wavelength   The distance in the direction of propagation for a wave to go through one complete cycle.

Wedge/Shoe   A device used to adapt a straight beam probe for use in a specific type of testing, including angle beam or surface wave tests and tests on curved surfaces.

Wrap Around Nonrelevant indications that appear on the CRT as a result of a short pulse repetition rate in the pulser circuit of the test instrument.

APPENDIX C

THREE-PLACE VALUES OF TRIGONOMETRIC FUNCTIONS							
Deg.	Sin	Tan	Sec	Csc	Cot	Cos	Deg.
0°	.000	.000	1.000	---	---	1.000	90°
1°	.017	.017	1.000	57.30	57.29	1.000	89°
2°	.035	.035	1.001	28.65	28.64	0.999	88°
3°	.052	.052	1.001	19.11	19.08	.999	87°
4°	.070	.070	1.002	14.34	14.30	.998	86°
5°	.087	.087	1.004	11.47	11.43	996	85°
6°	.105	.105	1.006	9.567	9.514	.995	84°
7°	.122	.123	1.008	8.206	8.144	.993	83°
8°	.139	.141	1.010	7.185	7.115	.990	82°
9°	.156	.158	1.012	6.392	6.314	.988	81°
10°	.174	.176	1.015	5.759	5.671	.985	80°
11°	.191	.194	1.019	5.241	5.145	.982	79°
12°	.208	.213	1.022	4.810	4.705	.978	78°
13°	.225	.231	1.026	4.445	4.331	.974	77°
14°	.242	.249	1.031	4.134	4.011	.970	76°
15°	.259	.268	1.035	3.864	3.732	.966	75°
16°	.276	.287	1.040	3.628	3.487	.961	74°
17°	.292	.306	1.046	3.420	3.271	.956	73°
18°	.309	.325	1.051	3.236	3.078	.951	72°
19°	.326	.344	1.058	3.072	2.904	.946	71°
20°	.342	.364	1.064	2.924	2.747	.940	70°
21°	.358	.384	1.071	2.790	2.605	.934	69°
22°	.375	.404	1.079	2.669	2.475	.927	68°
23°	.391	.424	1.086	2.559	2.356	.921	67°
24°	.407	.445	1.095	2.459	2.246	.914	66°
25°	.423	.466	1.103	2.366	2.145	.906	65°
26°	.438	.488	1.113	2.281	2.050	.899	64°
27°	.454	.510	1.122	2.203	1.963	.891	63°
28°	.469	.532	1.133	2.130	1.881	.883	62°
29°	.485	.554	1.143	2.063	1.804	.875	61°
30°	.500	.577	1.155	2.000	1.732	.866	60°
31°	.515	.601	1.167	1.942	1.664	.857	59°
32°	.530	.625	1.179	1.887	1.600	.848	58°
33°	.545	.649	1.192	1.836	1.540	.839	57°
34°	.559	.675	1.206	1.788	1.483	.829	56°
35°	.574	.700	1.221	1.743	1.428	.819	55°
36°	.588	.727	1.236	1.701	1.376	.809	54°
37°	.602	.754	1.252	1.662	1.327	.799	53°
38°	.616	.781	1.269	1.624	1.280	.788	52°
39°	.629	.810	1.287	1.589	1.235	.777	51°
40°	.643	.839	1.305	1.556	1.192	.766	50°
41°	.656	.869	1.325	1.524	1.150	.755	49°
42°	.669	.900	1.346	1.494	1.111	.743	48°
43°	.682	.933	1.367	1.466	1.072	.731	47°
44°	.695	0.966	1.390	1.440	1.036	.719	46°
45°	.707	1.000	1.414	1.414	1.000	.707	45°
Deg.	Cos	Cot	Csc	Sec	Tan	Sin	Deg.

APPENDIX D

Acoustic Properties of Materials

MATERIAL	DENSITY ρ=gm/cm³	LONGITUDINAL WAVES		SHEAR (TRANSVERSE) WAVES		SURFACE (RAYLEIGH) WAVES	
		VELOCITY V_L = cm/μs	IMPEDANCE Z_L = gm X 10²/ cm²-s	VELOCITY V_T = cm/μs	IMPEDANCE Z_T = gm X 10²/ cm²-s	VELOCITY V_R = cm/μs	IMPEDANCE Z_R= gm X 10²/ cm²-s
AIR	0.001	0.033	0.33	-	-	-	-
ALUMINUM 1100-O	2.71	0.635	1,720	0.310	840	0.290	788
ALUMINUM, ALLOY 2117-T4	2.80	0.625	1,750	0.310	868	0.279	780
BARIUM TITANATE	0.56	0.550	310	-	-	-	-
BERYLLIUM	1.82	1.280	2,330	0.871	1,600	0.787	1,420
BRASS (NAVAL)	8.1	0.443	3,610	0.212	1,720	0.195	1,580
BRONZE (P-5%)	8.86	0.353	3,120	0.223	1,980	0.201	1,780
CAST IRON	7.7	0.450	2,960	0.240	1,850	-	-
COPPER	8.9	0.466	4,180	0.226	2,010	0.193	1,720
CORK	0.24	0.051	12	-	-	-	-
GLASS, PLATE	2.51	0.577	1,450	0.343	865	0.314	765
GLASS, PYREX	2.23	0.557	1,240	0.344	765	0.313	698
GLYCERINE	1.261	0.192	242	-	-	-	-
GOLD	19.3	0.324	6,260	0.120	2,320	-	-
ICE	1.00	0.398	400	0.199	199	-	-
LEAD, PURE	11.4	0.216	2,460	0.070	798	0.063	717
MAGNESIUM, ALLOY M1-A	1.76	0.574	1,010	0.310	539	0.287	499
MOLYBDENUM	10.09	0.629	6,350	0.335	3,650	0.311	339
NICKEL	8.8	0.563	4,950	0.296	2,610	0.264	2,320
OIL, TRANSFORMER	0.92	0.138	127	-	-	-	-
PLASTIC (ACRYLIC RESIN-PLEXIGLASS)	1.18	0.267	315	0.112	132	-	-
POLYETHYLENE	-	0.153	-	-	-	-	-
QUARTZ, FUSED	2.20	0.593	1,300	0.375	825	0.339	745
SILVER	10.5	0.360	3,800	0.159	1,670	-	-
STEEL	7.8	0.585	4,560	0.323	2,530	0.279	2,180
STAINLESS 302	8.03	0.566	4,550	0.312	2,500	0.278	2,500
STAINLESS 410	7.67	0.739	5,670	0.299	2,290	0.216	2,290
TIN	7.3	0.332	2,420	0.167	1,235	-	-
TITANIUM (TI 150A)	4.54	0.610	2,770	0.312	1,420	0.279	1,420
TUNGSTEN	19.25	0.518	9,980	0.287	5,520	0.265	5,100
WATER	1.00	0.149	149	-	-	-	-
ZINC	7.1	0.417	2,960	0.241	1,710	-	-

D-1

APPENDIX E

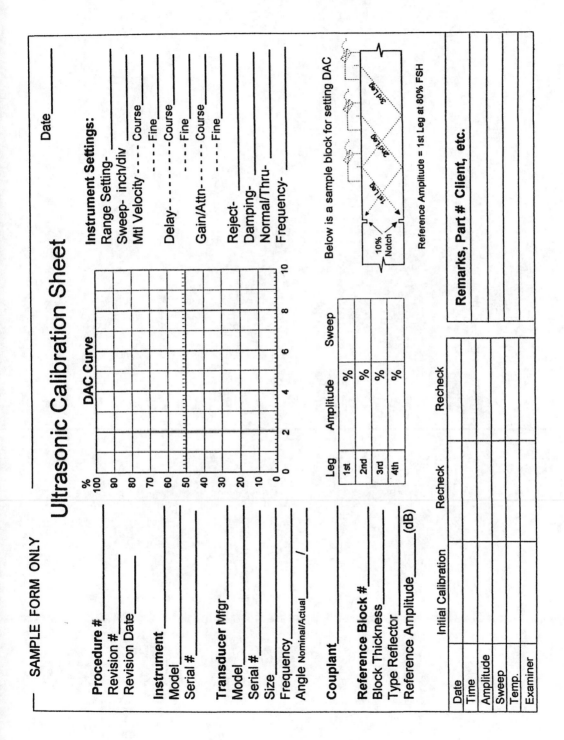

APPENDIX F

Angle Beam Examination Data Record

Job Number_____   Procedure Number_____

Drawing Number_____   Specification_____

Material_____   Reference Amplitude_____(dB)

Type_____   Scanning Amplitude _____

Average Part Thickness_____   Other_____

Indication Number	Scan Direction From − side From + side	Maximum % of DAC DAC From SDH or Notches	Sweep Reading Sound Path Distance	Surface Distance (+ or −) Exit Point to weld ₵	X Location (+ or −) ₵ to Indication	Y Location Inches from 0° Ref. and Total Length	Depth of Reflector Below the Surface

Notes:

Sketch cross section of weld if needed.

Inspector_____   Level_____ Date_____